88
Chinese
Medicine
Secrets

Visit our How To website at **www.howto.co.uk**

At **www.howto.co.uk** you can engage in conversation with our authors – all of whom have 'been there and done that' in their specialist fields. You can get access to special offers and additional content but most importantly you will be able to engage with, and become a part of, a wide and growing community of people just like yourself.

At **www.howto.co.uk** you'll be able to talk and share tips with people who have similar interests and are facing similar challenges in their lives. People who, just like you, have the desire to change their lives for the better – be it through moving to a new country, starting a new business, growing their own vegetables, or writing a novel.

At **www.howto.co.uk** you'll find the support and encouragement you need to help make your aspirations a reality.

How To Books strives to present authentic, inspiring, practical information in their books. Now, when you buy a title from **How To Books**, you get even more than just words on a page.

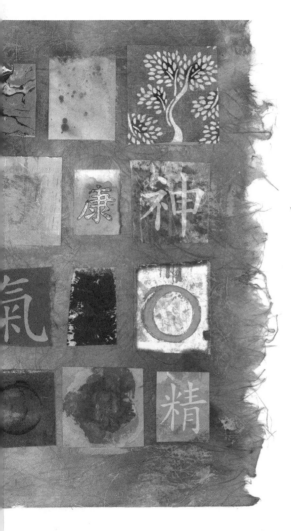

88
Chinese
Medicine
Secrets

How to cultivate

lifelong health,

wisdom and

happiness

ANGELA HICKS

howtobooks

Published by How To Books

Spring Hill House, Spring Hill Road,
Begbroke, Oxford OX5 1RX, United Kingdom
Tel: (01865) 375794, Fax: (01865) 379162
info@howtobooks.co.uk
www.howtobooks.co.uk

How To Books greatly reduce the carbon footprint of their books by
sourcing their typesetting and printing in the UK.

First published (as *77 Ways to Improve Your Wellbeing*) 2009
Second edition 2011

British Library Cataloguing in Publication Data
A catalogue record for this book is available from the British Library

ISBN 978 1 84528 430 5

Cover design by Baseline Arts Ltd, Oxford
Produced for How To Books by Deer Park Productions, Tavistock
Typeset by Kestrel Data, Exeter, Devon
Printed and bound in Great Britain by Bell & Bain Ltd, Glasgow

Contents

Chapter 5. Secrets of Balancing Work, Rest and Exercise   109

Chapter 8. Staying Healthy and Preventing Disease   **182**

Author's note

My thanks to everyone who has helped me to write this book.

First, my thanks to the practitioners and patients who have been so willing to talk to me about their experiences of acupuncture, herbs and making lifestyle changes.

Secondly, my thanks to the people who have read through this book and commented on it. Especially Judith Clark for her proofing and useful overview and Peter Mole, Matt Payne and Jane Serraillier for their helpful comments and suggestions.

Finally, my love and appreciation to my husband John, who supported and encouraged me throughout the time I was writing this book.

Please note that the organs and some other words have slightly different meanings when used in a Chinese medicine rather than a Western medicine context. With this in mind I have capitalized all Organs when they are used in a Chinese medicine context and used lower case if I am using them in a Western medicine context.

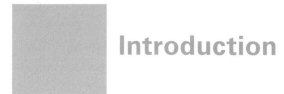

Introduction

I still remember when I first studied Chinese medicine. As I learnt parts of the theory about *yin* and *yang*, *qi* and the Five Elements my perspective on life was transformed and, over thirty years later I'm still fascinated – and healthy!

I found one particular part of the theory especially empowering. It was the knowledge of what causes disease and how we can remain healthy. Chinese medicine had a viewpoint about the prevention of disease that was totally new to me. It was sensible and down to earth and yet capable of changing lives.

Before studying Chinese medicine I had never really thought about why we become ill. I had assumed that some people were 'unlucky' and became unhealthy while others were lucky and managed to stay well. Health seemed to be a game of chance.

Times are changing. Thankfully many people now understand that there are underlying causes to their illnesses and that they can participate in their own wellbeing. At the same time there is an impending crisis within the medical profession. Deaths from cancer, strokes and heart disease are increasing. A stay in hospital seems to risk infection and the costs of the National Health Service are spiralling out of control. This is good reason for us to look after our own health and to keep ourselves well.

The Chinese have one of the few cultures that has preserved accurate knowledge about how to stay healthy. This lifestyle advice has been documented in a way that it is easy to follow. By following it we have a better chance of remaining well throughout our lives.

This book describes many of these useful ways in which Chinese medicine suggests we can keep ourselves well. It is written in the form of eighty-eight 'secrets'. Understanding these secrets will enable us to improve and maintain our health and prevent many illnesses in the future. I have also included modern research that backs up the Chinese view.

As a teacher and practitioner of Chinese medicine I often hear stories of patients who have improved their health enormously or who are now maintaining good health by changing their lifestyle. In this book I have drawn many examples from these people. Some people have gained this lifestyle advice from a practitioner. Going to a practitioner for treatment can be an important step when we are ill. These treatments can also help to maintain our health. But if we only have treatment 'done to us' and go back to the lifestyle that has made us sick, we may not stay well.

This book is for all of us who want to sustain our health. It provides guidelines to enable us to do so. I hope you too can receive the benefits that so many have enjoyed.

Good luck and good health!

1 You Can Be Really Well

You really can live longer!

Stunning results from research has found that people can extend their lives by up to 14 years by not smoking, drinking moderately, eating healthily and keeping physically active. A study surveyed 20,244 men and women aged between 45 and 79. Those who had smoked, drank, failed to exercise and had not eaten enough fruit and vegetables were four times more likely to have died during a period between 1993 and 2006 than those who didn't.[1]

In the 21st century people are becoming increasingly aware that there are many benefits to be gained from a healthy lifestyle. They realize that they can not only extend their lives and become healthier, they can also feel more contented and positive and have more vitality, stamina and clarity of mind.

Chinese medicine practitioners have observed and used the principles of a healthy lifestyle for thousands of years. As a general rule Chinese people have tended to place a higher priority on maintaining their health than have Western people.

A survey carried out by the office of Population Censuses and Surveys in England in the 1990s illustrates the benefits they gain from their attitude.[2] This research found that only 29% of Chinese pensioners have serious and long-lasting illnesses, compared with 36% of white people and 43% of people of Indian or Pakistani origin. These statistics are truly amazing – especially bearing in mind that most of the people included in this census were living in an unfamiliar culture. In China itself we would expect the results to have been even more spectacular.[3]

1

The *Nei Jing* or *The Yellow Emperor's Classic of Internal Medicine* is China's most famous medical textbook and contains advice about health and lifestyle. It was written in about 200 BCE. Since that time Chinese medicine has developed practical guidelines based on how lifestyle affected people's wellbeing. By paying attention to the way we eat, sleep, work and exercise as well as balancing our emotions, Chinese medicine practitioners were aware of what modern research is only just discovering. Lifestyle can have a huge impact on our health, happiness and longevity.

Chinese health 'secrets' were tried and tested over thousands of years. They have been passed down through families and have been quoted by the great Chinese doctors. As a result they are guidelines we can rely on and are quite different from various food and lifestyle 'fads' in the West.

Unfortunately the pressures of the 21st century often lead people away from a lifestyle that can benefit their body, mind and spirit. This book gives you Chinese medicine's profound yet simple guidelines to enable you to deal with these stresses.

What's in this for me?

There are many positive gains to be made from a healthy lifestyle. Table 1 gives some potential negative and positive effects. Although we can't avoid all diseases, we do know that every illness has a cause. The main causes of disease discovered by Chinese medicine over 2,000 years ago are still as relevant today. They form the chapter headings of the book and the first column in the table. Please be aware that this is just an overview and there are many more positive and negative effects that can be had.

Table 1. The positive and negative effects of a healthy lifestyle.

Lifestyle area	Unbalanced	Balanced
Constitution	Degeneration and ageing A painful and miserable old age Over-extending self leading to exhaustion	Youthfulness and longevity Vitality and vigour into old age Living within confines of constitution
Diet	Tiredness and lethargy Becoming overweight Food reactions and sensitivities Physical pains and discomfort Physical illnesses	Energy and vigour Staying slim A feeling of wellbeing Ease of movement Freedom from disease
Emotions	Anxiety and agitation Foggy mind Isolation and alienation Feeling miserable and overly serious Easily defeated Feeling stuck in a rut	Internal peace Mental clarity An ability to deal with intimacy A good sense of humour Emotional resilience Ability to use setbacks to grow
Work, rest and exercise	Poor health and tiredness Dissatisfaction and boredom Pain and stiffness Numbness of body and decreased awareness Tension and tight muscles Overweight and muscle wasting	Good health and vitality Fulfilment in work life Fluid and easy movement Increased consciousness and body awareness Liveliness, relaxation and calmness A slim and well-toned body
Climate	Succumbing to physical illnesses Inability to fight disease Pain, discomfort and immobilization Illness due to unseasonal activity	Freedom from physical illness Strong immune system Feeling of vitality and wellbeing Flowing and adjusting with the seasons

An ounce of prevention is better than a pound of cure

The consequences of an unhealthy lifestyle often take time to emerge and we can damage our health without knowing it. A bad diet or lack of exercise, for example, may take years before producing a symptom. The practice of a healthy lifestyle is important in order to prevent illness. Prevention means acting *before* the problems manifest.

Illnesses that are easily prevented

Some illnesses are easy to avoid with simple lifestyle changes. Here are two examples.

A colleague had a patient whose children had stomach pains. The patient wanted to bring them to have acupuncture treatment. This practitioner asked what they ate and was told that their diet included a lot of cold food such as iced drinks and ice cream. My colleague suggested that although treatment would be possible, they should first try reducing the amount of cold food the children were eating. The patient returned two weeks later and told him that they had taken his advice and were amazed because this simple solution had cured the stomach pains. Chinese medicine understands the effects of cold in the diet. You will find out more in Chapter 3 on diet and in Chapter 6 on the effects of the climate.

Most of us also make choices with regard to the balance of our work, rest and exercise. For example, if we work and don't rest for long periods then we can get worn out and may succumb to illnesses more easily. Illnesses such as chronic fatigue, frequent colds and flu, anxiety, tiredness, depression and many other conditions, may be due to returning to work before we are really better.

Recently a patient with chronic fatigue syndrome told me that she regretted not convalescing when she was ill with a severe infection. She returned to work before she was better and is now reaping the consequences. She realized that a change in her lifestyle habits would have prevented this illness.

Events we can't predict

Life will never be totally predictable, however, and other illnesses are less easy to avoid. Stresses like bereavement, accidents and other emotional traumas can't be avoided and can certainly take their toll on our health. We can compare a healthy lifestyle with an insurance policy. Good lifestyle habits will enable us to cope better through unexpected crises and help us to prevent illness in the future.

We've taken a glimpse at Chinese medicine in relation to illness. To understand the Chinese medicine view of health, we need to find out more about *qi*, which can be translated as energy.

Living a *qi*-enhancing lifestyle

Chinese medicine teaches us that our health is dependent on the balance of the *qi* (pronounced and sometimes written down as chi) in our bodies. *Qi* is our life force. When we have abundant *qi* that is flowing smoothly then we are healthy physically, mentally and spiritually. When our *qi* is deficient or blocked, we become unhealthy.

Although *qi* cannot be seen, it nevertheless penetrates every cell, allowing us to feel, think, move and have vitality. When we die the *qi* has left our body and the life force has gone. A lifestyle that enhances our *qi* will sustain our health. A lifestyle that weakens or blocks our *qi* will cause us to lose our health. We can decide between these two options.

The true 'pill' – lifestyle change

Practitioners of Chinese medicine look at the balance of each person's *qi* and view each individual as a whole – this includes their environment and lifestyle.

Most of us now know that lifestyle affects our health but we are still oriented towards a Western viewpoint of disease. If we have something 'wrong' with us, we expect a pill to take it away. When we go to a doctor they often feel obliged to hand us a prescription. If this doesn't work then we feel we haven't had the right thing 'done' to us.

In comparison, practitioners of Chinese medicine assess each individual as a whole and look for the cause of a person's problem. They understand that most Western medicines will only take away a symptom. The medicines will bring temporary improvement but won't deal with the underlying cause, so we can expect the symptom to return or a new symptom to appear later. Chinese medicine understands the true 'pill' – lifestyle change. We need to adapt our lifestyle to support our health and happiness.

Listen to your body

When we are ill we need to pay more attention to our health. In reality this is often when we feel least able to cope. We may take as many short cuts as possible. For example, eating 'fast' food makes our lives easier and many people are attracted to poor-quality foods when their *qi* is weak.

A friend recently commented that she noticed that if she was tense and stressed then she tended to eat fatty and sweet food like chocolate bars. The quality of these foods could further weaken her *qi* over a period of time. She then went on to say that if she gives herself the opportunity to do yoga or *qigong* (see page 133) and relax, then the desire to eat these foods goes away. She then ends up looking forward to eating a wholesome meal.

Ignoring the body's messages leads to illness and discomfort, while paying heed enables us to enjoy the benefits of health and happiness.

What will be the benefits?

All of us can benefit from some simple adjustments to our lifestyle. This can mean increased vitality, greater wellbeing or many of the other benefits shown in Table 1.

Improvements may be to do with current problems and many 'named' diseases can be affected. These may include digestive and bowel disorders, headaches, joint problems, mental and emotional complaints, circulatory disorders, gynaecological conditions, skin diseases, chest complaints and reproductive disorders, to name only a few. By modifying our lifestyle we can expect to feel healthier physically, mentally and spiritually.

If we are really ill it is always best to go to a doctor or a practitioner of Chinese medicine such as an acupuncturist or herbalist. Chinese medicine will increase our *qi* and help to restore our health. If we have treatment from a Chinese medicine practitioner this can then give us the strength to make necessary changes to our lifestyle. We can always benefit from living healthily and keeping ourselves well creates long-lasting changes in our health.

How to read this book

This book gives you secrets about all aspects of your life. You may want to read through each chapter in turn, then go back to try out one or two of the suggestions from the action boxes. Or you may wish to dip in and out of different sections trying the suggested actions as you go. Secrets 79–88 are useful tips about how to make lifestyle adjustments. Remember that it's important to change at your own speed – small changes can often have a major impact.

I'd like to remind you of two final points:

- **First, the process of change takes time**. Some changes take only a short time to carry out, but it may take years truly to integrate others into our lives. If we are patient with ourselves we may be surprised to find that we are making alterations quite effortlessly and find that we are naturally living a healthy lifestyle.

- **Secondly, we can't expect to be perfect**. Life is a process of growth and development and we can use our 'failures' as feedback for the future. Through trial and error we'll find out the best ways to live our lives to a healthy old age.

However you choose to use this book, I hope you gain much from learning about the Chinese wisdom that can nourish your life, and enjoy the next steps on your journey.

2 The Secret of Respecting Our Constitution

Our constitutional essence and long-term health

Why do some people lead an unhealthy lifestyle, yet stay well, whereas others need to look after themselves more carefully? The answer lies in a very well-kept secret. It is down to what Chinese medicine calls our 'constitutional essence'. Interestingly there is no equivalent concept for this in Western medicine. Understanding it can help us to deepen our awareness of our health and how to remain healthy.

Essence and our development

Chinese medicine says that we inherit constitutional essence (see Figure 1) from our parents. It is laid down when we are conceived and it creates our underlying strength and vitality. While we are in the womb this essence nourishes and sustains us. Once we are born, however, we are nourished by *qi* that comes from the food we eat and the air we breathe (for more on *qi*, see page 5).

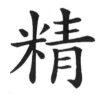

Figure 1. The Chinese character for constitutional essence (translated as *jing* in Chinese medicine). The left side of the character has four grains or seeds bursting forth. The right side signifies blue-green – the colour reminiscent of sprouting plants. The whole character implies that the essence that is stored in the Kidneys is the foundation of our energy and the seed of life itself.

Although after our birth we are maintained by *qi* from food and air, our constitutional essence still has an important role to play in our health. Constitutional essence is stored in the Kidneys and is responsible for the cycles that allow us to grow, reproduce and develop. The fact that we develop normally from babies to children is due to our essence. It then helps us to move through puberty and on to adulthood. Constitutional essence allows us to be fertile and for women to give birth. Later on, the female or male menopause indicates that our essence is declining.

If we conserve this constitutional essence we can remain strong, vigorous and healthy well into old age. If this essence is depleted the drying-up process of ageing will progress more rapidly. We may also have increased susceptibility to ill-health.

Essence as a reservoir

Our constitutional essence is like 'sap' or 'juice' that we can draw on during a crisis or periods of overwork. It acts like a reservoir of energy. If we look after our health by eating well and balancing work, rest, exercise and sexual activity, then our reserves will remain fully stocked and we won't need to draw on them. They might even be topped up by some of the *qi* which is formed from the food we eat and the air we breathe. If we overdo it, however, we will deplete our reserves of this essence. When the constitutional essence becomes depleted, this can result in us feeling exhausted and easily becoming ill. This sap-like substance gives us the healthy glow and moistness we have in our youth. Long-term depletion can cause us to become dried up, lose vigour and age prematurely.

By learning to assess the strength of our essence, how we deplete it, how to conserve it and how we can replenish and improve it, we can positively affect our quality of life. In this chapter we will discuss these secrets of preserving our constitutional essence.

1 Conserve your constitutional essence

Some of us are born with what seems to be an infinite amount of constitutional essence. Others start off with less. We can compare this with a car battery. Some cars have larger batteries than others. No matter what its size, a car battery needs to be looked after. If people frequently forget to switch off their car lights or other accessories the battery can go flat. Sensible drivers look after their batteries. Our constitutional essence is like our own internal battery. Some of us are careful and conserve it. Others use it recklessly. Unfortunately, it is easier to replace a car battery than our essence.

The father of a friend of mine is still vigorous even in his late 80s. His hair didn't turn grey until his mid-eighties and he only started to feel he was getting a little old when he was 81! He has always led a healthy life and he ate fresh food from his garden at every meal. He had a desk job but would take a brisk walk for 40 minutes every day and at weekends he enjoyed sporting activities.

In comparison another friend survived on very little sleep, was nearly an alcoholic, had too much sex and spent most of his time partying in his late teens. At the age of 20 he collapsed completely and stayed in bed for almost a year being nursed by his mother. He is now in his mid-30s and has recovered, but still has to be careful to sleep and eat regularly. If he overdoes it he becomes exhausted and gets backache. In spite of being a healthy child he drained his batteries at an early age.

Ways in which we deplete our constitutional essence

Our supply of constitutional essence is finite. Those born with a plentiful supply are considered lucky! Some people who are born with a strong constitution don't realize this, however, and think they have an infinite supply of energy as my friend above did. Those who have a smaller car battery are often more careful with themselves. In the end they can outlast the people who started life with a larger battery but didn't look after it. These are some of the ways we might use up our constitutional essence:

- overwork

- not enough sleep

- too much sex

- too much exercise or over-activity

- poor diet or irregular eating habits

- severe and/or continual long-term stress

- long periods of dissatisfaction or emotional instability

- long-term severe illness

- long-term drug or alcohol abuse.

Most of us are born with a 'normal' amount of this essence – although we can never have too much. If we have normal constitutional essence but are depleting it, the first symptom we might experience is excessive tiredness. Although we can't restore the constitutional essence we've used up, if we don't ignore the symptoms of depletion and we rest, we can improve the quality of what we have left and top it up with *qi* acquired from living a healthy lifestyle.

Action Box

Take few minutes to consider how well you are caring for your constitutional essence. Write two lists. In the first list write down what lifestyle activities you do that conserve your essence. In the second write down what you do that might deplete it. Remember how you are supporting yourself by doing the things written in the first list. Now think of anything you might change from the second list to help to conserve it more.

Remember that change takes time and you can start by making very small changes. The following secrets will give you some other ways to help you to conserve your essence.

2 Assessing your constitutional strength

Chinese medicine gives us guidelines that help us to check our constitutional strength. The main ways to measure this are by assessing:

- signs of premature ageing

- physique and stamina

- the strength of the jaw

- the ears and earlobes.

Signs of premature ageing

People who are healthy and can recover from illnesses and stress relatively well usually have a normal amount of constitutional essence. There are two ways that depletion occurs. Some people are born with a depleted constitutional essence. Living unhealthily can also deplete it. The essence is used up as we age.

The signs of depleted essence are those associated with premature ageing. This 'juice' or 'sap' is drying up. Symptoms include premature greying hair, hair loss or baldness, drying skin and wrinkles, brittle bones, tinnitus (ringing in the ears), losing teeth, dizziness, backache, constant colds, difficulty conceiving, poor concentration and memory, extreme tiredness, an early menopause in women or impotence in men.[1]

When people are born with a constitutional essence deficiency there may be a delay to the normal stages of their development. Infants may start walking or talking late and develop slowly or the onset of puberty may be delayed. Another sign is that people might continually fall ill.

Physique and stamina

Another useful way of assessing the strength of our constitution is to consider our overall stamina. If we are very robust, have a naturally strong physique and can easily work hard and recover our energy quickly, this may indicate that we have strong constitutional essence.

Those people who have a strong constitution may sometimes fail to understand the fragility of the rest of the population who have weaker or even normal constitutional energy. They may wonder why others can't just 'pull themselves together and get on with life'. A person with strong constitutional essence will easily recover from illness.

If we have an abundant supply of constitutional essence, we should still be careful. Our constitutional essence is finite and, if we overdo it, we too can end up exhausting ourselves. Those frailer people who are looking after their health now might fare better in the future.

The strength of the jaw

A large head on a strong broad jaw line is indicative of someone who has been born with a healthy constitution. According to Chinese facial diagnosis, the jaw and lower part of the face relate to the later years of a person's life. This can be used as an approximate guide to how we will fare in old age. A strong jaw indicates that we will have a long life, remain healthy into old age and easily recover from illness. A weak jaw indicates poorer health.

We can observe the ear and the jaw line to assess roughly how we will deal with illnesses later on in life. If both are of good size and shape we should fare well. If not, we might start to prepare ourselves now and build up our constitutional essence in order to have a healthy future.

The ears and ear lobes

Ancient Chinese texts talk about the size of the ears and the length of the earlobes as a guide to the strength of the constitutional essence. The ears should be well placed – that is, not too high on the head. They should also be a good size in relation to the person's build. The earlobes should also be long.

If we look at Oriental pictures of the Buddha, he is often depicted as having huge earlobes – perhaps signifying the extraordinary strength of his essence. Long and full lobes are said to indicate a strong constitution; small thin earlobes are said to indicate a less strong one.

Action Box

If you are ageing well, are relatively healthy, have a good physique and are robust, congratulations! You probably have strong or normal constitutional essence. Make sure you look after it by reading the lifestyle suggestions in the rest of this book! You may also have a strong jaw and long ear lobes which are additional indicators of your good health.

If you don't see these characteristics when you look in the mirror, make sure you are not being too self-critical. You probably have a more 'normal' supply of essence like the rest of us and need to ensure you look after your health.

3 Accept your limits and live within their confines

Whether our constitutional essence is strong, normal or slightly below par, we can benefit from the advice below. These are four guidelines that will help us live within the limits of our constitutional essence.

1. Work within your capacity and listen to your body's needs

Nowadays many people think it's normal to overwork. Often they override their exhaustion and keep active instead of resting. Once we are in the habit of overworking it becomes difficult to stop. There is often conflict between the needs of family and work. I often tell patients that listening to the body is the key to maintaining health. It can take time to train ourselves to notice our body's signals, which may be tiredness, feeling low or simply being 'out of sorts'. At first we may prefer to ignore them. The more we can tune in and take notice, the more we can make healthy adjustments to our lifestyles.

2. Avoid comparing your capacity with someone else's

If we notice that we are less robust than others it's best to accept the situation and work within our limits. If we expect to be like friends or family members who have a very strong constitution we will always find ourselves wanting. If we work on our health steadily and then compare ourselves with ourselves, we will value our own accomplishments rather than someone else's. We can, for example, look at how much we've improved compared with one or two years ago. This will enable us to feel proud of what we have done and help us to get the best from our lives.

3. Charge your batteries now

Our health is our insurance policy. Many people take their good health for granted. If a crisis arises out of the blue, we can deal with it better if our batteries are fully charged beforehand. If our batteries are already going flat we may be left completely depleted afterwards. When we are depleted, we are more vulnerable to illness. Even if we think we have loads of energy and vitality, a healthy lifestyle will keep it that way rather than depleting us when we most need it.

4. If necessary, restore your strength with Chinese medicine

Acupuncture and Chinese herbs can boost our energy, stamina and wellbeing. These treatments recognize the need for tonics. Unfortunately, there are very few tonics left in Western medicine. Western medicine can remove individual symptoms but doesn't usually deal with the underlying cause or restore our overall energy.

Action Box

Here is a summary of the four guidelines that will help us live within the limits of our constitutional essence:

1. Work within your capacity and listen to your body's needs. Your signs and symptoms are signals that you are out of sorts – don't ignore what your body is telling you.
2. Avoid comparing your capacity with someone else's. Value your own accomplishments rather than continually looking at other people's.
3. Charge your batteries now. If you think your constitutional essence is even slightly depleted, now is the time to act. By acting now to restore it, you are buying insurance for your future health.
4. If necessary restore your strength with Chinese medicine. A change in lifestyle may be difficult to undertake when you are unhealthy and lacking in energy. If necessary you can embark on a course of Chinese medicine treatment to improve your health. If you are depleted and unwell this can enable you to gain the strength you need in order to make lifestyle changes that can support your health in the future.

 # Important transformation times that can change your life

Chinese medicine understands that the constitutional essence moves in seven-year cycles in women and eight-year cycles in men. Every seven or eight years there are shifts in our body, mind and spirit during which transformations occur. These affect our physical and psychological health. If we take special care of our health during these transformation periods we can end up feeling rejuvenated and healthier. If, on the other hand, we ignore them, we may become less well.

There are four special times when our health can substantially change for the better or worse. They are:

1. puberty
2. leaving home

3.   pregnancy and childbirth
4.   menopause.

Puberty

According to Chinese medicine theory the seven and eight-year cycles lead to puberty in girls at around the age of 14 (2 × 7 years) and for boys around the age of 16 (2 × 8 years). When I was 13 or 14, my girlfriends and I noticed that we had suddenly grown tall, were developing breasts and were maturing physically and emotionally. At the same time the boys were less developed. Then a few years later the boys suddenly shot up (usually around 16 years or 2 × 8 years), grew tall and became very attractive! The age gap was due to the girls having a seven-year cycle and maturing two years before the boys.[2]

Some people blossom when they come into puberty. Others find that it is a difficult time from which they never truly recover. Recently it has grown to be almost a 'norm' for some teenagers to abuse themselves with drink, drugs, poor food and lack of rest. Teenagers think they will live forever! Those who have strong constitutional essence probably come through unscathed but we are seeing the results in the teenagers who are less constitutionally strong.

Mental diseases such as schizophrenia are more common – especially in teenage boys. Problems of long-term obesity can set in at an early age. Other physical illnesses such as heart attacks and strokes are now occurring at younger and younger ages. We can't stop teenagers from doing what they will do but we can let them know that their constitutional essence is finite and precious and hope that some will take notice.

Leaving home

Many people leave home in their late teens or early twenties. It used to be the time when people got married. Now this transition time is often when young people go to university or set up home with a partner. If this is a good move and the young person has a lot of support and help, the mental adjustment from dependence to independence runs smoothly and the young person moves on to being a self-sufficient adult. If leaving is a struggle it can take a toll on our health. Depression and instability can occur and a negative cycle can be set in place.

Pregnancy and childbirth

In the next secret we will discuss this transition in more detail and how traditionally in Chinese society women have looked after themselves by 'doing the month' after giving birth.

Pregnancy is a very important shift for men as well as women. During the initial period after birth a man can feel estranged from his partner for a while – the baby has taken his place! After about six months he will usually find himself reconnecting with his wife as the baby learns that she or he isn't the centre of the world and both parents start to participate and feel more involved with childcare.

Menopause

Menopause occurs in women at around the age of 49 (7×7 years). A lot of women feel unwell throughout this time and hot flushes and anxiety are often seen as a 'norm'. It is interesting that the signs and symptoms of menopause were the exception rather than the rule at one time in Chinese society. This is changing as China 'modernizes' and comes more into line with Western culture.

Conversely for those women who look after themselves or have strong constitutional essence menopause can be the beginning of the healthiest time of their lives as they develop from a mature adult into a 'wise woman'. (For more on the male 'menopause', see Secret 7 page 25.

5 'Do the month' after pregnancy

The constitutional essence is a baby's main source of nourishment while it is in the womb. Pregnant women who don't rest or take care of themselves may find their reserves begin to become depleted – nature dictates that the baby will take whatever it needs. This could result in women developing signs of essence deficiency leading to illness and later premature ageing. Some common symptoms found during pregnancy are, for example, hair loss, backache, weakened teeth and extreme tiredness – all symptoms of essence deficiency.

By taking care of themselves during and after pregnancy women may find these symptoms are less severe and then rectify themselves more rapidly once the baby is born. Mothers who have many pregnancies close together may also become depleted.

On the other hand, as you will see below, women who have looked after themselves during and after pregnancy may end up healthier than before they became pregnant.

'Doing the month'

Rest is particularly important immediately after giving birth. At this time a woman in China is said to 'be in the month'. During this period she rests completely. All her needs are taken care of – traditionally by her mother-in-law (nowadays this may be your partner, a good friend or hired help).

As well as resting, she eats plenty of meat, especially chicken, to strengthen her, avoids getting emotionally upset and, as she has been temporarily weakened by the process of giving birth, she also avoids the effects of Wind and Cold (see Chapter 6).

'Doing the month' and our health

In a study of over 100 Chinese-American women in California, those who were questioned said they considered 'doing the month' was beneficial to their health. Most thought women who don't rest after giving birth would suffer 'grave consequences' for their health later on. These might be illnesses such as poor energy, joint problems, infections and depression. Other well-known symptoms are ageing skin, greying hair, breaking nails and poor-quality teeth.

'Doing the month' and post-natal depression

Interestingly, the study found that women who 'do the month' don't expect to get post-natal depression. This idea didn't make sense to the Chinese-American women questioned. This is in contrast to women in Western countries who often take it for granted that they will suffer from depression after childbirth.

A period of rest after giving birth used to be a normal part of Western post-natal treatment. Nowadays many women in the West no longer regard this as necessary. Women often leave hospital soon after having a baby, and although their energy is still depleted, they go back to 'normal' life almost immediately. Many of our role models encourage us to 'get up and go' after giving birth rather than recovering our energy.

The consequences of not, 'doing the month'

Interestingly Chinese tradition states that if a woman does not 'do the month' and subsequently becomes ill there is only one way she can restore her health – to become pregnant again and this time to 'do the month' properly![3] We might decide we do not want to take this course of action! It does, however, underline the seriousness with which Chinese women took their health during pregnancy.

Action Box

If you are pregnant or considering it, you might have thought about looking after yourself during the pregnancy, but what about after giving birth? A month resting is the best option. For some people a whole month is too much. If you can't manage a complete rest you might consider how you can get support in order to rest as much as possible. Remember that time spent looking after yourself after the birth can set you up for good health in the future for you and the baby.

Motherhood is a time when women can blossom and improve their health – or a time when they can lose it. Parenthood can also be an important turning point for both mother and father as they care for and nourish their newborn infant.

 6 Looking after the affairs of the bedroom

When I was first studying acupuncture I went to a seminar led by a well-known Chinese doctor who lived in New York. He skilfully diagnosed patients and suggested treatments. Many of the patients were very ill and each patient was given an individual diagnosis and treatment. There was only one statement that he made to almost everyone. It was: 'Don't have too much sex.'

In the West today the benefits of sex are widely publicized. It is understood that enjoying a satisfying sex life helps us to remain in close and fulfilling relationships. When we are ill or tired, however, we might consider making some temporary changes in order to regain our health.

Constitutional essence and sexual activity

Chinese medicine notices that the quality of male sperm reflects the strength of the constitutional essence. During orgasm men lose a small amount of this essence and deplete the Kidneys where it is stored. Although this seems to apply slightly more to men, who lose sperm when they ejaculate, it does also apply (to a lesser extent) to women.

The Chinese doctor I mentioned earlier said: 'After a man has had an orgasm he needs to rest for a day. After a woman has had an orgasm she needs to rest for a few minutes!' This may have been said with tongue in cheek but it nevertheless illustrates the point. You may think it is unfair that women get off so lightly but as you saw in the previous secret, women deplete their essence too but more during pregnancy and childbirth.

Sex and ill-health

When we are well, it is healthy to have an active sex life. When we are ill, we need to cut down to help us to regain our health. Most people naturally have less desire to have sex when they are ill or overworking and this is normal. Many feel that they *should* have more sexual appetite and deplete themselves trying to have a 'normal' amount of sex. Others try to please a partner who has greater desire.

A sympathetic partner will understand that the lack of desire is a sign of ill-health or a different constitution and not of rejection. Once health is restored sexual desire usually returns. One member of a couple having a lack of sexual desire can, however, be a source of great friction. This is especially true after the birth of a baby or during chronic illness and compromises may need to be made.

'Too much' sex

Some people react differently. When they are tense and overworked they have a heightened desire for sex. They may find tension can be released through orgasm. In this case they may be engaging in too much sexual activity which may be temporarily satisfying but in the long term may drain them. This can produce a vicious circle that is hard to break. They initially get tense because they are stressed and tired but ultimately become more tired and stressed due to too much sex. In this situation the person needs to deal with the underlying causes of the tension. One important sign of having too much sex is a dull backache around the Kidneys where the constitutional essence is stored.

The importance of sex

The benefits of sex are also important. Sexual closeness is, of course, a way to create intimacy within a relationship and this will lead to better health. As long as it is not used habitually, sex can also be an important way to release tension. When people have tight muscles, orgasm can relax them and may free up blocked energy and even cure pain. Frustration, which can build up through a lack of sexual activity, can be just as damaging to our health as too much sex.

Action Box
Age and sex

As well as giving us guidelines about sexual activity when we are unwell, Chinese medicine books discuss what constitutes a normal sex life at different stages in our lives. All the ancient Chinese doctors had different opinions, however!

In general it is normal for younger people to enjoy a more active sex life and for this to decline steadily, as a person gets older. As a rule of thumb, a maximum frequency of ejaculation for a man in good health could be as follows:

- 20 years old, twice a day.
- 30 years old, once a day.

- 40 years old, every three days.
- 50 years old, every five days.
- 60 years old, every ten days.
- 70 years old, every thirty days.

This should be halved if the person is unwell or tired.[4]

It is best that our sexual activity also changes with the seasons. It is normal to enjoy more sex during the summer when it is hotter and have less sexual activity in the colder months.

The male menopause is not what you think!

Recently it has become fashionable to discuss the male as well as the female menopause. Although it is true that men do have a menopause (or andropause) it is not at the same time as the female menopause.

The seven and eight-year cycles discussed above have been described in the *Nei Jing* or *Yellow Emperor's Classic of Internal Medicine*, one of the oldest Chinese medicine classics. Women's cycles end at around 49 year (7 × 7 years) when their fertility declines. A man's cycle, however, goes on until 64 or 65 years (8 × 8 years). This is when men retire from their traditional role as the breadwinner. At this time their whole life can shift. If men adjust well to this major lifestyle change they can go on to a happy and healthy old age. If they don't adjust well, it can lead to premature ageing, a loss of their role and status and possibly severe illness or even premature death.

8 Strengthen your constitutional essence by breathing into the *dantien*

As well as ensuring that we eat healthily and have enough work, rest and exercise, Chinese medicine suggests that we can improve the quality of the essence by activating an area approximately four fingers' width below the umbilicus called the *dantien*. This is both a centre of gravity and balance in the body and a useful focal point for breathing.

Breathing into the area of the dantien or belly breathing is also a useful way to relax. When we are tense we start to breathe high up into the chest. It is impossible to be stressed if we breathe low down into the belly.

Action Box

Breathing into your dantien

Natural deep breathing into the lower abdomen relaxes us and this in turn builds our energy. To breathe into the lower abdomen, breathe in through the nose and at the same time allow the lower abdomen, sides and back to expand. Then breathe out and allow them to relax. Some people find it helpful to imagine a balloon expanding and contracting in this area. Breathing in this way is natural and easy. At the same time it will move the area of the lower abdomen and activate the *dantien* (see Figure 2).[5]

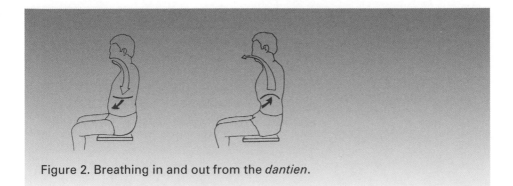

Figure 2. Breathing in and out from the *dantien*.

9 Strengthen your constitutional essence by sensing into the *dantien*

The Chinese call the *dantien* 'the seat of constitutional essence'. By practising Chinese exercises such as *qigong* or *tai ji quan* we can improve our vitality and wellbeing and become more relaxed. We can also strengthen the quality of our constitutional essence and strengthen our Kidney *qi*.

Sensing into the *dantien* is a simple yet effective way to strengthen and activate it. Both adjusting our posture so that our centre of gravity naturally falls into the *dantien* and focusing our attention on it can enable us to do this. The action box below shows us two different ways to sense into this area.

Action Box

Adjusting your posture

For the basic qigong standing position, stand with the feet facing forward and shoulder width apart. Bend the knees slightly so that they are unlocked. Relax the hips and lower abdomen and allow the weight to travel down to the arches of the feet. Allow the pelvis to curl slightly forward so that the lower back is straight. Relax the shoulders and neck and let the arms hang loosely at the sides. Keep the head upright and look straight ahead.[6]

27

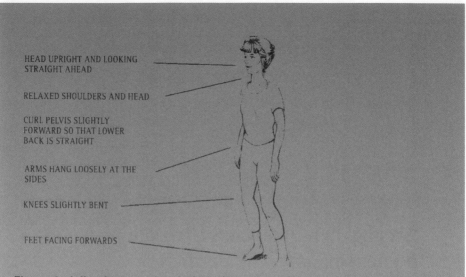

HEAD UPRIGHT AND LOOKING
STRAIGHT AHEAD

RELAXED SHOULDERS AND HEAD

CURL PELVIS SLIGHTLY
FORWARD SO THAT LOWER
BACK IS STRAIGHT

ARMS HANG LOOSELY AT THE
SIDES

KNEES SLIGHTLY BENT

FEET FACING FORWARDS

Figure 3. Adjusting posture during *qigong* exercises

A *qigong* exercise for focusing attention on the *dantien*

As well as focusing our attention on the *dantien*, this exercise can aid our concentration, strengthen our *qi* field to help ward off infections and enable us to develop the ability to direct our *qi* both inside and outside our body:

1. Stand in the basic standing posture pictured above.
2. Imagine that your *qi* is extending outwards from your *dantien*, in all directions. Some people find it helps to imagine their *qi* as a white light, others just get a 'sense' of the energy.
3. As the *qi* expands, feel your arms and hands slowly moving outwards. Expand your arms wider and wider until you are reaching out to the universe.
4. Feel your energy is extended to the universe and at the same time notice you can remain centred in your lower abdomen.
5. Now allow the *qi* from the universe to contract. As it comes in allow it to move your arms inwards until the *qi* is in your *dantien* and is getting smaller and smaller but never disappearing.

Repeat for 5–10 minutes continuing to allow the *qi* to expand and contract.

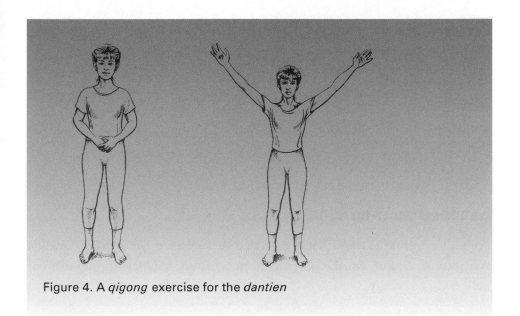

Figure 4. A *qigong* exercise for the *dantien*

3 Dietary Secrets

Eat food as medicine

Chinese medicine teaches that a balanced diet ensures our physical, mental and spiritual health. On the other hand poor eating habits will diminish our wellbeing and energy.

Chinese people are far more aware of their diet than many Westerners are. Over many years I've asked Chinese students, practitioners and friends, 'How important is food to you?' They proudly tell me that they are passionate about their food and diet.[1]

As children many Chinese people were taught about the unique qualities of different foods – foods for longevity, foods to cool them down, foods to heat them up or foods to balance their *yin* and *yang*. As they grew up they found that food is not only an enjoyable pleasure, but also a source of good health. There is an ancient saying in Chinese medicine that 'food and medicine come from the same source'.

Chinese dietary advice is different from Western nutrition. It is more holistic. Although Chinese medicine practitioners understand the importance of carbohydrates, proteins and fats, vitamins and minerals, they equally understand that the balance of food proportions and the taste and temperature of food are a part of the whole concept of dietary health.

If we change the quality and quantities of the food we eat on a daily basis it can have a profound effect on our health. It might also prevent some major illnesses commonly found in the West. Research has found that conditions such as coronary heart disease, cancers such as stomach, colon and breast cancers, gallstones, high blood pressure, goitre, diabetes, osteoporosis and arthritis are all related to a typical Western diet.[2]

In the West our present diet has deviated far from that eaten by our ancestors. It is hardly surprising that so many of our current health problems are exacerbated by a poor diet. A research paper written on the health of the elderly states that: 'People are often unaware of how much the national diet has changed during the last decades. We can now afford to eat foods every day that our ancestors only had on festive occasions.'[3]

In this chapter we will be looking at the most significant areas of the Chinese diet. This will help us eat healthy and enjoyable meals – just as our ancestors once did and as do those who keep these ancient secrets alive today.

10 Balance the proportions of your food

The typical proportions of a Chinese diet are similar to the diet that our ancestors ate in the past. It can be divided into three main groups in these quantities (see Figure 5):[4]

- 40–45% vegetables, as well as some fruit.

- 40–45% grains and carbohydrates – the Chinese typically eat a large amount of rice and in the north they mainly eat millet.

- 10–20% of rich foods such as meat, fish, seafood and eggs, dairy products, fats and oils and sugars.

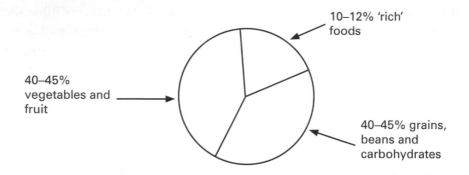

Figure 5. Proportions of food in a well-balanced diet.

As the West has grown more affluent we have changed the proportions of food we eat until our 'normal' diet has been turned on its head. Westerners now commonly eat a diet containing a large amount of rich foods that have strong tastes. We often eat only a small proportion of the grains, beans and vegetables that should be a staple part of our diet.

Chinese medicine considers richer foods, such as animal products, dairy products and other fats, to be 'special' and extremely nourishing – but only in small quantities. Excessive amounts of these foods are harder for our digestion to assimilate. Eaten in large quantities they will end up upsetting our digestion and the balance of our health.

Has there ever been a time when we have eaten more in line with these correct quantities? We can go back to the 1940s when British people were eating a rationed wartime diet. The occurrence of coronary heart disease and many other illnesses were at an all-time low during this period. Comparing the average British diet in 1948 with more recent years we now eat 50% more meat and twice as much cheese, but less than half as much bread, potatoes and other carbohydrates – an astonishing difference![5] The British diet in wartime was much closer to the Chinese diet than it is now.

A diet based on grains and vegetables is central to most cultures. Two other well-researched diets are the Japanese diet[6] and the Mediterranean diet.[7] These diets were carefully measured during the 1960s and both use similar proportions to the typical Chinese diet. The life expectancy for Greek people who ate this diet during the 1960s was among the highest in the world.[8] At the same time the rates of many cancers, coronary heart disease and other diet-related chronic illnesses were at their lowest level, despite far more limited medical services than those available today.[9]

The United States Department of Agriculture[10] and the British Health Education Authority[11] (along with the World Health Organization) now recommend a diet using quantities of foods similar to those eaten by the Chinese.

Action Box

Write down a list of all the food you ate and drank yesterday. Take an objective look at this list. How did the proportions approximately compare with the following?

- 40–45% vegetables, as well as some fruit.
- 40–45% grains and carbohydrates.
- 10–20% of rich foods such as meat, seafood and eggs, dairy products, fats and oils, and sugars.

If you want to make a more accurate assessment, carry a notebook around with you and write down everything you put into your mouth for the next week. Note down *all* food and drink – including any snacks. This is a useful exercise for two reasons:

1. You will have a clear overview of your overall dietary intake for a week.
2. You will find your diet naturally improves as you do this.

Is there any improvement needed? If so, what might you do? It is best to make small, simple adjustments. Don't try to make too many changes at once.

Keep this list to hand when considering suggestions in the rest of this chapter.

11 Rely on 'economical' foods in your daily diet

Great importance is given to grains, as well as vegetables, in a typical Chinese diet. As far back as the Tang dynasty, between 582 and 682 CE, Sun Si Miao, a famous physician, wrote that the medical function of diet should not be neglected. He advocated eating a simple, healthy diet. He said: 'One should cut down on quality food and rely on a diet of economical food.'[12] To him 'economical food' was grains and vegetables, and 'quality' food, richer food such as meat.

The Chinese word for food is *gu*, which means 'grain'. Chinese medicine considers that the *qi* or energy in our body is originally created from the food we eat combining with the air we breathe. The initial *qi* manufactured from food is called *gu qi*. *Gu qi* goes through a 'rotting and ripening' process via our Stomach and Spleen[13] until it becomes very refined and usable by our body as 'true' *qi* – which nourishes our Organs and gives us vitality and wellbeing.

Grains and beans should form about 40–45% of our diet and should be eaten daily. The staple food of Chinese people is, of course, rice. To achieve variety rice can be combined with other grains such as wheat in breads and pastas, as well as with oats, rye, buckwheat, amaranth, quinoa, couscous and millet.

We should, however, be careful about eating too much wheat. Many people in the West overdose on it and eat it for breakfast, lunch and dinner. As wheat is a very 'dampening' food (as opposed to rice which clears dampness from the body) it should be eaten in moderation and not to the exclusion of all other grains. (There is more about damp on pages 40 and 159).

Dried beans such as soya beans, and other soya products such as tofu and miso[14] can supplement grains. Beware of some processed soya products such as soya milk and soya yoghurt, however. These have been much publicized as an alternative to dairy products but are not fermented in the same way as tofu and miso and can be difficult to digest. It has been reported that these more processed soya products can cause thyroid and other problems.[15] (See page 61 for substitutes.)

Other beans such as lentils, split peas, aduki beans, black-eyed beans, chickpeas (garbanzos), mung beans, haricot beans and kidney beans can also be used. All grains and beans should be as unprocessed as possible and, like all other foods, organically grown whenever available. (See the Action Box for cooking methods for grains and beans).

Action Box

Cooking grains and beans

Listed are the basic cooking methods for commonly used grains and beans. Measure using a standard teacup or mug, keeping the same size throughout the recipe. These amounts serve three to four people.

Grain (1 cup)	Liquid	Cooking time	Notes
Rice	2 cups	30 mins	Keep the lid on and do not stir the rice.
Barley	3 cups	1½ hours	Soak first for 15 mins. Stir occasionally. Use in soups and stews or as a breakfast cereal.
Millet	3 cups	20 mins	Roast in a pan until it is browned before boiling. Use as a side dish or in soups and stews.
Couscous	2½ cups	10–15 mins	Cover with boiling water and leave until water is absorbed. Can be used as a side dish.
Amaranth	1½ cups	20 mins	Can be used as a breakfast cereal.
Quinoa	2 cups	25 mins	Rinse well before cooking to remove bitter taste. Can be used as a porridge or in soups and stews or as a side dish.
Buckwheat	1½ cups	10 mins	Also good in pancake mixes or breads.
Oat (flakes)	2 cups	10 mins	Used for porridge or in baking.
Rye	4 cups	1 hour	Use in casseroles and stews.

All beans, except lentils and split peas, need to be soaked overnight. This cuts the cooking time and is said to remove any gas from them. Do not add salt until they have finished cooking as salt prevents them from becoming tender. Beans can be eaten by themselves or mixed in a dish with rice or other grains. These amounts serve three to four people.

Bean (1 cup)	Liquid	Cooking time	Notes
Aduki, black-eyed or kidney	3 cups	1½–2 hours	Soak overnight first. Simmer until soft.
Chickpeas or haricot beans	3 cups	1–2 hours	Soak overnight first. Simmer until soft.
Soya beans	3 cups	3 hours	Soak overnight first. Simmer until soft.
Split peas or lentils	2 cups	30–45 mins	No need to soak.

12 Choose vegetables – full of rich, life-enhancing *qi*

Vegetables, along with some fruits, should provide at least 40–45% of our daily food intake. Vegetables are probably the most neglected part of the Western diet. Some people, especially young teenagers, can go for days without eating any plant products at all. This is potentially damaging to their health.

Between 1966 and 1982 a study was carried out in Japan on 270,000 people. The participants in the study ate colourful vegetables such as carrots, tomatoes, chicory, spinach, broccoli, leeks, turnip leaves and pumpkins every day. The results of this study found that merely adding vegetables to the diet substantially reduced the risks of cancers, heart disease and many other terminal illnesses. At the same time ageing slowed down by a huge 10–15 years! Fatigue was also considerably lessened, as were stress disorders such as insomnia and irritation.[16]

Many other studies have researched the reduced risk of many cancers and other diseases from eating vegetables and fruit.[17]

It is only a small change for us to increase the amount of vegetables on our plates. Studies show that the long-term ramifications could be considerable when we make this simple switch – especially if our vegetables are well prepared.

Action Box

Cooking vegetables

Steaming and stir-frying are two popular and healthy ways of cooking vegetables.[18] Roasting and boiling are two other methods that can be used. If you regularly use only one method of cooking vegetables, perhaps try another for variation.

Steaming

This is considered to be the most neutral and harmonious way of cooking vegetables (and many other foods used in the Chinese diet). It is fast, preserves nutrients and maintains the natural flavour of the vegetables. You can use either a Chinese steaming basket or a good-quality metal steamer.

- Chop the vegetables and place them in the steamer.
- Add the water to the pan. It is important that the water doesn't touch the vegetables.
- Simmer until the vegetables are tender, which should take about 10 minutes. Make sure the water doesn't evaporate.

You can keep the remaining broth for a soup or use it as a warm flavourful drink.

Stir-frying

Stir-frying is, of course, a traditional way of cooking many foods in China. This method also preserves the colour and flavour of the vegetables. A wok, which is a round-bottomed pan, is most often used, although a large frying pan can be just as good:

- Wash, then slice all the vegetables into small pieces of an approximately even size. Make sure they are not too wet.
- Pre-heat the wok and then add oil (about 2–3 tablespoons).
- Once the oil is hot add the densest vegetables, such as carrots and broccoli, first.
- Begin stirring the vegetables as soon as they go into the wok.
- Once all the vegetables are in and partly cooked, turn the temperature down, cover the pan and simmer for about 5 minutes until the vegetables are fully cooked (the aroma will tell you they are ready). The resulting vegetables will be crisp, nutritious and juicy.

Roasting

This is simple and nutritious and preserves vitamins and minerals. It is especially good for root vegetables such as carrots or parsnips:

- Place the vegetables in a baking dish and cover with oil.
- Add any flavouring such as salt, pepper or garlic.
- Place in an oven pre-heated to 180 °C/350 °F and leave to cook for 30 to 45 minutes until the vegetables are tender.

Boiling

Boiling is the easiest means of cooking vegetables but does tend to destroy some of the nutrients:

- Place the vegetables in half to one inch of water.
- Cover the pan and simmer for about 10 minutes. You can try simmering vegetables in stock for added flavour.

After boiling vegetables, the water can be used as a basis for stock or to add to gravy to improve the flavour.

13 Avoid too much raw and cold food

Chinese people are often shocked and mystified when they see people in the West happily eating raw food and vegetables. They would suggest that vegetables should be lightly cooked before eating. There are two main reasons for this.

First, raw vegetables are harder to digest than cooked ones. Cooking starts to break down food and aids the Stomach's digestive processes. This will result in more nutrients being absorbed. For example, only 50% of a carrot will be absorbed if it is eaten raw, compared to 65% when cooked.[19]

Secondly, and very importantly, practitioners of Chinese medicine understand that the process of digestion requires heat. The Stomach can be compared with a large cooking pot full of soup at boiling point.[20] Putting large amounts of cold food into this soup will cool it down substantially and so require more energy to break it down. Over a long period eating raw vegetables and cold food can make us very lethargic due to the extra energy we need to digest it.

I recently advised a patient to cut down on cold foods. I was surprised when he came back and thanked me, saying he'd always preferred warmer foods but thought salads were healthy so had forced himself to eat them. He was not unusual. Many people eat salads and drink iced drinks throughout the winter. On a hot summer day a salad or cold drink can be very satisfying but we need to eat in accordance with the temperature of the seasons.

Our ancestors recognized the importance of eating warm food. One traditional adage is that we should eat at least one hot meal a day. Many of us have now forgotten this sensible piece of advice and eat cold food throughout the day, even in the middle of winter. Adding at least a hot soup to our diet and lightly cooking our vegetables can make a substantial difference.

Action Box

Think about the foods you have eaten recently (either from the list you made from the Action Box on page 33, or just what you have eaten today) and consider:

- Is there a balance of hot and cold foods in your diet?
- Do you eat according to the season or not? For example, do you eat salads in the winter?
- Do you eat according to your temperature? For example, do you easily feel cold but still continue to eat raw and cold foods?
- Do you routinely drink iced drinks, even when you are cold?
- Do you eat food straight from the fridge without allowing it to warm up first?

Don't overdose on 'rich' foods

Meat, fish, poultry, eggs, dairy produce, fats and sugars are all classed as 'rich' foods in Chinese medicine and should be eaten only in small quantities. Good-quality animal products, dairy products and oily foods are very nourishing but they only need to form 10–15% of our diet.

We can compare eating large amounts of these rich foods with taking ten times the prescribed dose of a medicine. We might think that a larger dose will improve our health by ten times as much as a normal dose – but of course we will really be taking a dangerous overdose.

Action Box

Think about the foods you have eaten recently (either from the list you made from the Action Box on page 33, or just what you have eaten today) and consider:

* What percentage of the food you commonly eat comes under the bracket of 'rich' food?
* Are you eating too large or too small a percentage of these foods?

Also see below the list of phlegm or damp-forming foods. These are also rich foods.

15 Know your phlegm and damp-forming food

The most famous Chinese medicine classic, the *Nei Jing*, written 2,000 years ago, says: 'Heavy and greasy food causes a change that may induce illness.'[21] One result of overdosing on rich food is the formation of 'phlegm' and 'damp' in our system. Symptoms can include bloating and bowel disorders such as loose bowels, as well as chronic blocked sinuses, phlegm in the chest, heavy limbs, achy joints and one common problem of our time – obesity. A lack of concentration, tiredness, a muzzy head or even depression can also occur.

Action Box

If you recognize that you have some of the above symptoms and suspect you have phlegm and damp, the following foods may exacerbate your condition.

Some of the most common damp and phlegm-forming foods are:

* dairy produce – milk, butter, cheese, cream, etc.
* fatty foods including fatty meat and fried foods
* sugar and sweeteners
* wheat – in excess – including breads and pasta
* excessive amounts of concentrated juices such as orange juice, tomato puree
* excessive amounts of peanuts, bananas
* excessive alcohol.

You might notice that many (although not all) of these foods are 'sticky' in nature. We can start to notice the varying effect different foods have on our system.

Sometimes *reducing* rather than completely cutting out these foods will help to clear our system, but in other cases – especially if phlegm and damp easily form in our systems – it may be best to cut these foods from our diet completely, at least for a while.

If you need to stop eating certain foods it is always best to substitute healthier alternatives. For some suggestions, see page 61.

Dairy produce in excess is phlegm and damp forming for most of us. People sometimes worry that they'll succumb to osteoporosis or become deficient in calcium if they cut down on dairy. This is not necessarily the case. The Chinese and Japanese have lived healthily on a diet containing little or no dairy produce for thousands of years. It is also ironic that the countries with the highest milk consumption (USA and Scandinavia) have the highest incidence of osteoporosis in the world.[22]

One of the best ways of preventing osteoporosis is regular weight-bearing exercise such as walking, running, cycling, swimming, playing racquet games or dancing.[23] Chinese exercises such as *qigong* or *tai ji quan* can also be beneficial. More is written about these exercises in Chapter 5.

16 Lose weight effortlessly!

Many people in the West find it difficult to lose weight and obesity has reached epidemic proportions. In China, people who eat a traditional diet rarely have a weight problem as their diet nourishes the Stomach and Spleen.[24]

The Stomach and Spleen are the two main organs of digestion and they are in charge of assimilating, moving and transforming our food and drink. Eating food that weakens these two organs often causes weight problems.

If we follow the suggestions below as well as the rest of the dietary suggestions in this chapter, we will naturally reach a healthy equilibrium in our weight:

- Eat nourishing food but avoid dieting. A nourishing diet contains grains and beans with fresh vegetables and fruit. If these are taken in the correct proportions they will strengthen the Stomach and Spleen and allow them to work at maximum capacity.

- Eat three meals a day regularly. Skipping meals weakens the Spleen.

- Cut down on damp and phlegm-forming food. These rich foods are sticky and difficult to digest and put a strain on the Spleen and Stomach (See page 40). Many people find that they effortlessly lose weight when they cut down on or cut out wheat.

- Avoid cold foods and drink. This can be a major cause of weight problems. Cold slows movement down, while heat speeds it up. Taking foodstuffs such as iced drinks, frozen yoghurts or too many raw vegetables will slow the metabolism.

- Avoid eating too much overly sweet food. The sweet taste is associated with the Spleen. A moderate amount of the sweet taste is very strengthening but an excess will weaken the Spleen. It is best to cut down on extremely sweet-tasting food and best to avoid food sweetened with white sugar altogether.

- Start doing moderate exercise. When we cut down on food the body thinks there is a famine and starts to conserve our food and energy. To lose weight we need to exercise, which will speed up the metabolism.

Action Box

A summary of ways to lose weight effortlessly:

- Eat nourishing food but avoid dieting.
- Eat three meals a day regularly.
- Cut down on damp and phlegm-forming food.
- Avoid cold foods and drink.
- Avoid eating too much overly sweet food.
- Start doing moderate exercise.

---

17 Be an 'almost' vegetarian

There has been much discussion over the years about whether it is healthier to be a meat-eater or a vegetarian. Chinese medicine suggests that we should eat only a small amount of meat because of its 'rich' qualities, which I have already mentioned. Research bears out this view.

Too much meat

Eating a lot of meat can lead to a diet that is far too high in fat. Studies have been carried out in the West on the correlation between a regular high consumption of meat in the diet with coronary heart disease and many types of cancer. Research carried out in the United States found a difference between people who consumed meat daily and those who didn't. Those who ate meat every day were found to have a 60% greater chance of dying from coronary heart disease than those who consumed meat less than once a week.[25]

Not enough meat

On the other hand, a lack of meat can lead to serious deficiency. A study has linked eating meat during pregnancy with healthier babies. In this study 549 women were surveyed between 1948 and 1954 and the offspring traced 40 years later. This research suggests that women who cut down on eating meat during pregnancy could risk producing children who suffer from an increased risk of high blood pressure and heart disease in middle age.[26]

Nourishing our 'Blood' by eating meat

Chinese medicine says that animal products such as meat and fish are especially effective for nourishing the 'Blood' in our bodies. It views Blood in a slightly different way from Western medicine. Blood is responsible for 'nourishing and moistening' our systems and for keeping our 'spirit' settled in the body.

If we become 'Blood deficient' we can have symptoms such as anxiety, panic attacks, insomnia and a poor memory. These are symptoms affecting our spirit. Other symptoms such as tiredness, cramps, pins and needles, light-headedness, dry skin, or floaters in front of the eyes can arise. This is because our system is not properly nourished and moistened by our Blood.

From these symptoms we can realize that Blood deficiency causes many disabling symptoms. These include anxiety, jumpiness and possibly a lack of confidence. A condition sometimes treated as a mental or emotional problem can simply be due to a deficient diet.

Action Box

Eating an 'almost' vegetarian diet

Chinese medicine recommends a compromise between vegetarianism and eating meat, in the form of an 'almost vegetarian diet'. We don't need to eat too much animal protein but a little will benefit our health. We only need to take 50–100 g/2–4 oz of animal products three or four times a week. The Chinese often cut their meat, fish or poultry into small strips and mix it with their rice or noodles.

· Sally's indecision about eating meat

Sally, who is 42 and a speech therapist, became convinced that she and her son needed meat in their diet. Both of them now feel the difference. Here she tells us what happened:

I went for acupuncture treatment as I had no reserves of energy left. With treatment I recovered my energy to a certain level but I always had to go back for more treatment every six weeks because my energy would crash down again. My practitioner said that my diet was the major factor stopping me from getting better. My husband and I had been vegetarian for 20 years and our children had never eaten meat. At first my practitioner's words didn't wash at all but I eventually changed my mind when my son Paul, who was coming up to 15 years, was also having problems.

At 15 he was under six stone, not tall and not going into puberty. He was also somewhat anorexic in his attitude to food. My practitioner said this might also be due to a lack of meat. Paul now eats meat two or three times a week with no comment and he's grown much taller and gone into puberty. He no longer looks as if he could be blown away by a puff of wind. Before he was having trouble going through GCSEs but now he's worked relatively hard for months without getting stressed at all.

I now eat meat too and it's made a huge difference – my tongue has actually changed colour! It was always very pale, now it's a healthy red and I can hardly recognize it as mine.[27] I was always a wishy-washy person and as a child I was thought to be anaemic, though blood tests showed that I wasn't. I now feel much stronger generally and feel fitter and I'm enjoying life more. I've even taken up tennis. In terms of treatment I now need much less. I went for a check-up in June then didn't go back until September and I was fine.

18 If you are vegetarian – be a well-balanced one

You may not want to eat meat on moral grounds. If this is the case then it is important to eat a vegetarian diet that is as well-balanced as possible. Here are some 'dos' and 'don'ts' for vegetarians:

- Don't substitute meat with cheese or other dairy produce as this does not create a well-balanced diet – cheese and dairy products are extremely rich foods.

- Try not to binge on sugary and fatty foods to make up for the lack of animal products and protein in the diet. The result of this can be huge shifts in mood and also weight gain.

Ensure that you are eating adequate amounts of protein and 'Blood'-nourishing foods:

- Include plenty of grains in your diet and combine them with beans and pulses.[28]

- Eat more protein substitutes. Two important ones are tofu and miso. Both are made from fermented soya and are very nourishing. Another substitute is Quorn. This is made from a fermented fungus mixed with egg white.

- Eat lots of seaweed products. Some common ones are hiziki, nori and wakame. Seaweed is commonly eaten in the Orient, although more by the Japanese than the Chinese. It is very nourishing, low in fibre and contains many minerals such as potassium, calcium, magnesium and iron as well as iodine (see action box for cooking instructions).

- Eat sprouted beans. Bean sprouts are considered to be energy-enhancing foods (see page 68).

- Eat plenty of dried fruits such as dates, apricots and figs to strengthen the Blood.

- Eat lots of vegetables, especially leafy green vegetables.

- Follow the suggestions in this book for balanced proportions in the diet.

Action Box

Simple ways to cook seaweed

Seaweed is traditionally used in the Orient, most commonly by the Japanese. It is especially useful for vegetarians to enrich their diet as it is rich in minerals. Here are basic recipes for some common types of seaweed, which are usually available from health/wholefood shops.

Wakame
Wash thoroughly. Use a piece one inch square per person. Add to cold water and soak for 5 minutes. Chop to the required size. Add to soups and stews, or it can be eaten alone or with vegetable dishes.

Hiziki
This is a tasty black stringy seaweed. Wash thoroughly then soak for 1 hour. Squeeze out the water and save it. Fry in a little oil for a few minutes. Add the soaking water and simmer until tender. This can be eaten alone or sautéed with vegetables like carrots or onions.

Kombu
Wash thoroughly. Use a piece one inch square per person. Soak for 15 minutes. This can be cooked with beans to tenderize them and prevent gas.

Nori (also known in the West as Laver)
This comes dried, in thin sheets. It can be toasted over a flame and then sprinkled on food or can be dipped into cold water and wrapped around rice to make rice balls.

Arame
Wash thoroughly. Use an amount the size of a ping-pong ball for two people. Fry with onions or soak for a few minutes then add to casseroles or stews.

47

19   Take good-quality food

We all know the expression 'You are what you eat'. Chinese medicine emphasizes how true this is. If we eat high-quality food it will be transformed into good-quality *qi* and Blood. This nourishes us physically, mentally and spiritually. The result is that we can begin to glow with good health. If we eat poor-quality food it lowers our vitality and the quality of our *qi* and Blood will be deficient. Over time this will result in ill-health.

Much of our food is now contaminated. Hormones and antibiotics are injected into animals and pesticides are sprayed on vegetables, dangerous preservatives and 'taste enhancers' are sometimes added to our food, and our air is polluted too. Genetically modified (GM) foods have been introduced into the food chain. These may all be having a profound effect on our long-term health. Unless we are eating organic foods we are now eating these pesticides, preservatives and drugs on a daily basis. Many people are increasingly aware that the human race cannot disturb nature without detrimental effects.

The BSE crisis in the UK in the 1990s was one example of the damage caused by interfering with nature. Other effects from long-term use of chemicals are bound to become more apparent in the years to come.

Problems arising from tampering with our foodstuffs are relatively new and are not, of course, mentioned in old Chinese texts. There is an increasing body of evidence that GM foods have a negative impact on the environment as well as on those who eat them. The best advice for us to follow is to eat simple, natural foodstuffs which are in season and grown around us if possible. These are the foods that our ancestors ate on a daily basis.

Organic foods

Nowadays the most unadulterated foods are ones we grow in our own gardens, or organically grown food. All food should be processed as little as possible.

Organic vegetables, fruit and meat products are now widely available and many of us are eating them as the majority of our daily diet. There is an increasing body of evidence that organic vegetables contain more vitamins and minerals than their non-organic counterparts.[29] They have the added advantage of tasting better as well as being healthier. Organic meat may be more expensive, but eating smaller amounts can make up the cost. Organic meat is much less likely to have chemical residues and the animals won't have been raised on GM feed.

What to eat if you can't buy organic

Non-organic vegetables have usually been treated with pesticides. There are over 100 types of pesticides, many including organophosphates, on the market. These can permeate the leaves and roots of vegetables and can't be removed just by rinsing. Pesticides are known to be extremely toxic and have been linked to low sperm counts and cancer.[30]

Vegetables and fruit have often been sprayed many times with different chemicals and a small proportion of samples come out above the limits when tested by monitoring agencies. A much larger proportion contain lower residues. No one knows the cocktail effect of these chemicals together and if there is an additional effect on those also taking medicinal drugs.[31]

Francis Blake, Standards Director at the Soil Association, also suggests:

> Carrots are the main root vegetable affected by organophosphates. The carrot root fly is difficult to treat and damage to the carrot makes it unsaleable. For this reason farmers use insecticides in the soil. Swedes can also be affected. The least affected root vegetables are beetroots, parsnips and celeriac, although none are totally clear of pesticides.

> Leafy vegetables may be better than root vegetables but consumers should be aware that nitrites in the soil will concentrate at the heart of leafy vegetables so it is better to eat the outside leaves of non-organic vegetables. These also contain the most vitamins and minerals.[32]

> ### Action Box
>
> If you can't afford organic vegetables, or you are eating out, you can at least eat the least polluted or least polluted part of vegetables. Likewise, you may decide that eating fish dishes may be a safer option in a restaurant – the seas are polluted but at least the fish haven't been injected with hormones! A patient I spoke to recently eats meat only at home. This ensures it's organic. If she goes out to eat she only eats vegetarian produce. However, organic meat is becoming much more common in restaurants – always ask where it has come from and who has certified it.

20 Avoid 'spoiled' foods

The Chinese call food that is no longer fresh 'spoiled' food. Cooked food that is more than 24 hours old loses some of its vitamins and minerals, but more importantly it begins to also lose its *qi* content. I've already mentioned that Chinese medicine teaches us that if we eat well we gain *qi* from our food. Over recent years the West has created another kind of 'spoiled food' that was unknown to the ancient Chinese. This is food that has very little *qi* content due to irradiation, preservatives and other added chemicals and also by using cooking methods such as microwaving.

> ### Action Box
>
> In order to enhance our *qi* it is best to eat food that is as fresh, pure and alive as possible. A useful rule of thumb when choosing food is: 'If it can't go off, don't eat it. If it can go off, only eat it when it's fresh.'

21 An enjoyable diet is the most nourishing

Another significant factor in our diet is enjoying our food. If we smell a really tasty dish cooking it activates our salivary glands and we start to feel hungry. Our saliva then helps to break down the food we put in our mouth.

After the food reaches the Stomach it can be 'rotted and ripened' more easily and we then get more *qi* and nourishment from it. If we don't enjoy our food we won't salivate and we won't digest it properly.

The Chinese call the smell of a stir-fry in the first few minutes as it comes from the cooking wok, '*Wok hay*' or '*Wok qi*'. This is the prized 'breath' from the food that is not to be missed.[33] To start to eat after the *wok qi* has disappeared is unthinkable for Chinese people who take pride in wholesome cooking. Presumably one reason for this is that it activates the salivary glands.

If we enjoy our food it will be easy for us to make nourishing meals. But what if we find it hard to build up an appetite for the food we are eating?

A rich diet that includes food such as chips, burgers and ice cream can become addictive. A diet high in vegetables and grains can at first seem extremely boring in comparison. A rich diet can be hard to give up but we can get caught in the trap of feeling guilty if we don't manage to stick to our new healthier routine. Guilt is as harmful as a poor diet.

Action Box

Sometimes the only food available to you may not be particularly healthy or nourishing. For example, you're away from home or work at lunchtime and can only find a burger bar. If this is the case, decide to eat with relish and *as if it is nourishing* – at least your mental state will then be positive and help you to gain the best possible nourishment from it.

Many people have ingenious ways of making their diet more enjoyable. For instance, a friend who changed to a healthier diet allowed himself a treat of one 'old style' meal per fortnight. He noted that after a few weeks the pasta, rice and vegetables seemed to be tastier than his previous food. He still allows himself a treat every so often and knows he can have an occasional coffee or chips if he wants them.

A patient who was strongly motivated to eat well for her health put more effort into making her food look attractive. We eat with our minds as much as with our bodies and producing tempting-looking food was a way to entice herself to eat better.

Regularity is also important. If we eat regular meals we start to get hungry whenever it is time for a meal, thus allowing ourselves to enjoy our food more.

Whatever way you choose, it is important to make your diet enjoyable as well as healthy. If you are eating a diet that is not appetizing you won't stick with it.

Remember that it takes about a month really to alter your habits. Once you have made the adjustments for several weeks they are more easily integrated into your daily life.

Simon's diet

Simon is 35 and enjoys his job as a sales rep because he drives all over the country. He has headaches and complains of feeling lethargic and tired much of the time. He sleeps well but often finds it hard to get up in the morning. The headaches come on every three or four days and are located on his forehead. His head feels heavy and the headaches are often worse after lunch. When he is stressed the headache can be all over his head and he feels as if his head will burst. This is the food he eats on a normal day:

8.00   *Breakfast*: A bowl of cereal with plenty of full-cream milk and sugar. A cup of coffee.

11.00   *Break at a cafe*: Cup of coffee and cake.

1.00   *Lunch*: A good fry-up at a motorway cafe – sausage, egg and chips. Apple pie and a cup of coffee.

3.30   *Break*: Cup of coffee and a cream cake.

5.00   *Stop on way home*: Cup of coffee.

9.00   *Evening meal*: After arriving home at 7 p.m. Pasta with a creamy sauce and vegetables with a piece of fruit. Cup of tea.

Simon's dietary problems

Simon's main problems are his high fat and dairy intake and too much coffee. The fatty food and dairy produce has put a strain on his Stomach, Spleen and Liver and have caused him to form damp in his system. The damp has caused him to feel heavy and lethargic. The damp is also causing the headaches. The coffee will irritate the Stomach and Liver and make his headache worse. He is eating late at night, straining his Stomach which will be digesting food late. He is getting some fruit and vegetables but not enough. It won't be easy for him always to eat well but he can look for the healthiest alternatives. His stressful lifestyle, driving to different parts of the country, is also contributing to his health problems.

Suggestions for Simon

- **Cut down on fat.** Change to a non-dairy 'milk' on cereal or have porridge. Choose less fatty options to eat at meals out if possible – there are usually some low-fat meals available. Have non-creamy sauces on the pasta or other dishes eaten in the evening.

- **Cut down on coffee.** Change to coffee substitutes when at home, take alternative hot drinks in a flask or drink mineral water at room temperature.

- **Eat as wholesome a diet as possible.** Try to eat more fresh vegetables and fruit when out at lunch. Many restaurants offer them. Eat other grains such as rice in the evening.

- **Arrange to eat earlier in the evening.** Simon and his wife share the cooking. He can arrange to cook on the days he gets home earlier.

- **Do some gentle exercise in the morning or during the day.** Simon is leading a very sedentary life and needs more exercise. Some *qigong* or other exercise in the morning will get his energy moving before he drives off for the day.

22 Know the temperature of your food

An important aspect to do with our diet is choosing food at a correct temperature and taste. These are secrets that have been kept well hidden from the West. We'll start by looking at the fascinating area of temperature.

Chinese cooking at its most excellent demonstrates how to combine warm, neutral and cool foods. Some foods are cooler in their make-up and others are warmer. This is not dependent on whether the food has been heated up or frozen but is rather something about its inherent nature. Foods are divided into 'hot', 'warm', 'neutral', 'cool' and 'cold'. Below is a list of some foods in the different temperature categories.[34]

Hot
Black pepper, butter, chicken fat, chillies, chocolate, cinnamon bark, coffee, crispy rice, curry, dried ginger, ginseng (Korean), lamb, onions, peanut butter, sesame seeds, smoked fish, trout, whisky, white pepper.

Warm
Barley, beef, beer, black-eyed beans, brown sugar, caraway, chamomile, cheese, chestnuts, chicken meat, chives, dates, egg yolk, garlic, fresh ginger, ginseng (Chinese), green (bell) pepper, ham, kale, kidney beans, leeks, lobster, miso, molasses, mussels, oats, parsley, parsnips, peaches, pomegranates, potatoes, prawns, quinoa, raspberries, sage, shrimps, soya oil, squashes, sunflower seeds, thyme, turkey, turmeric, vinegar, walnuts, wine.

Neutral
Aduki beans, apricots, beetroot, black tea, bread, broad beans, brown rice, buckwheat, cabbage, carrots, cherries, chickpeas (garbanzos), corn, egg white, ginseng (American), grapes, honey, hot water, kidney beans, lentils, milk, olive oil, oysters, peanuts, peanut oil, peas, plums, pork, raisins, red beans, rosehips, rye, salmon, soya milk, sugar (white), sweet potatoes, turnips.

Cool

Alfalfa sprouts, almonds, amaranth, apples, asparagus, barley, broccoli, cabbage, cauliflower, celery, chicory, corn, fish, mangoes, millet, mung beans, mushrooms, oranges, pears, pineapples, radishes, rhubarb, salt, seaweed, soya beans, soya sauce, spinach, strawberries, tangerines, wheat, wheat bran, wild rice.

Cold

Bananas, bean sprouts, cucumber, duck, grapefruit, green tea, ice cream, kelp, lettuce, peppermint, salt, seaweed, sorbet, sugar cane, tofu, tomatoes, water melons, yoghurt.

It is best to choose from the neutral foods for the largest percentage of our diet. If you notice that you tend to feel more cold or hot during the day or night you might bias your diet towards eating slightly more heating or cooling foods according to your temperature. The temperature of food can also be changed according to the season and you can eat warmer foods in the winter and cooler ones in the summer.

Action Box

We can balance the temperature of our food by combining warm and cool foods. When we eat warmer foods we can balance them with a food from the cooler section and vice versa. For example, tofu and other soy products are quite cooling in nature. Adding a little ginger, which is a heating food, can make them more warming. Lamb, which is very hot, is traditionally combined with mint sauce to cool it down. Vegetables are generally cooling, and meat is more heating. Eat these with a grain, such as rice, which is neutral, to create a very balanced meal. Interestingly salt and pepper, the two most used condiments in the UK, balance each other. Salt is cold and pepper is hot.

23 Not *too* hot or cold – keep it balanced

Cool or warm food should be taken in slightly lesser quantities than neutral food. Foods that are *very* hot or cold should be taken in only small amounts as they may have too extreme an effect. Large quantities may cool us down or heat us up too much.

Cooling or cold food

Fruit is a good example of cooling food. Not surprisingly many fruits that are cooling in nature grow in a more tropical climate. Tangerines, oranges, pineapples, bananas, melons and grapefruit are pleasant treats especially in hot weather when they have a cooling effect. They should not, however, be taken in large quantities in cold weather.

Too much cold food can cause symptoms such as loose bowels, profuse urination, stomach aches or period pains. Over a long period they could also make us feel tired through weakening the Stomach and Spleen.

Some people think that large quantities of fruit juice, such as orange juice, is a healthy option. However, drinking just one glass of orange juice is similar to eating 8–10 oranges in one go and can be extremely rich as well as cold.

We should always bear in mind what foods are in season and where they are grown. Locally grown food that is in season is always our best choice.

Warm and heating foods

You might notice that many meats and fatty foods such as butter, chicken fat, lamb, beef and peanuts are more heating in nature. We know that these are nourishing in small quantities but they should not be taken in large amounts.

Large amounts of heating foods can make us restless, irritable and angry and could give us symptoms such as high blood pressure, headaches, palpitations or constipation.

Action Box

Consider the foods you have eaten recently (either from the list you made from the Action Box on page 33, or just what you have eaten today). Divide them into five groups by putting them, to the best of your ability, into the following sections:

Hot
Warm
Neutral
Cool
Cold

- Are most of the foods on your list in the warm, cool and neutral categories?
- Or are there a lot of extremely cold or hot foods?
- Is the overall balance of the foods biased more towards either heating or cooling foods?

If you are eating a balance of warm, cooling and neutral foods, the temperature of your diet is fairly well balanced.

If you are eating more cold and hot foods, or if your diet is biased towards either cold and cooling or hot and warming foods, without being balanced by the opposite temperature, then your diet is not so well balanced.

By including more foods of a less extreme temperature in your diet you will be eating in a more balanced way – and this is likely to have a positive effect on your health.

24 Blend the tastes of your food

Including a variety of tastes in our diet ensures that it is healthy and balanced, and also keeps our food interesting. Chinese medicine divides the tastes into five different categories: bitter, sweet, pungent, salty and sour. Each of these tastes will affect us in different ways and all food has one or a combination of these tastes. You may notice, for example, that a radish is both bitter and sweet, while garlic is salty and pungent. These affect the functioning of the corresponding Organ, as shown below.

Bitter (Heart and Small Intestine)

Alfalfa, asparagus, beer, broccoli, celery, chicory, coffee, grapefruit rind, lettuce, radishes, raspberry leaf tea, turnips, vinegar, watercress.

Bitter foods slightly cool the body and are used to stimulate the digestion. They can also be used to cool fevers and to clear bowel problems, which are due to heat. Because of their purging action they should only be used in small quantities in our diet if our energy is deficient.

Sweet (Stomach and Spleen)

Aduki beans, apples, apricots, barley, beef, beetroot, cabbage, carrots, celery, cheese, cherries, chicken, chickpeas, coffee, courgettes (zucchini), corn, cucumber, dates, grapes, grapefruit, honey, kidney beans, lamb, lettuce, malt, mandarins, milk, mung beans, mushrooms, oats, oranges, peaches, peanuts, pears, pineapples, plums, pork, potatoes, radishes, raspberries, rice, spinach, strawberries, sugar, tomatoes, walnuts, wheat, wine.

The sweet flavour described in Chinese medicine is subtle. It is different from the strong sugary taste that is often used in the West. Sweet is probably one of the most frequent tastes found in foods – note the number of foods listed in the category above. The sweet taste affects the Stomach and Spleen. In Chinese medicine these Organs have the function of transforming all of our food and drink in order to nourish us. If taken in the correct quantities, sweet foods such as rice, chicken, cabbage and carrots will have a strengthening effect.

Extremely sweet foods in large quantities will weaken the Stomach and Spleen and have a dampening effect. People frequently crave chocolates and sweets because their Stomach and Spleen are deficient. This can become a vicious circle. The more depleted these organs become the more we crave sweet foods. The Stomach and Spleen then correspondingly become even more feeble. This will result in very deficient *qi* in our whole system or even malnutrition.

Pungent (Lung and Large Intestine)

Black pepper, cabbage, cayenne pepper, cherries, chillis, cinnamon, cloves, cumin, garlic, green (bell) pepper, horseradish, leek, marjoram, mint, mustard, nutmeg, peppermint, radishes, rosemary, soya oil, turnips, watercress, wheatgerm, wine.

Pungent foods are sharp and acrid tasting and their effect is to disperse and move obstructions in the *qi* and Blood. Like Bitter, they should be taken in small quantities by those who have very deficient energy.

Salty (Kidney and Bladder)

Barley, crab, duck, garlic, ham, kelp, lobster, millet, mussels, oysters, pork, salt, sardines, seaweed.

The Salty flavour is commonly found in seaweed and seafood. This taste acts as a diuretic and will clear excess water from the system. Frequently people are advised to avoid salt in their diet and it is true that it is best not to take an excessive amount. This is especially the case if a person retains fluids and has weak Kidneys, which are the organs associated with this taste. A small amount of salt can be beneficial, however, if a person has too much moisture in the body.

Sour (Liver and Gall Bladder)

Aduki beans, apples, apricots, blackberries, blackcurrants, cheese, crab apples, gooseberries, grapes, grapefruit, green leafy vegetables, lemons, lychees, mandarins, mangoes, olives, peaches, pear, pineapples, plums, pomegranates, raspberries, sour plums, strawberries, tangerines, tomatoes, trout, vinegar.

Finally, Sour foods have the opposite effect to Pungent ones. They stop discharges and are astringent in their action. They help problems such as urinary incontinence, diarrhoea or excessive sweating.

Action Box

Balancing tastes

In general it is best to include all the flavours in our diet without eating any of them in excessive amounts. If we crave a certain taste this may indicate that the associated Organ is out of balance. A small amount of a food may enhance the functioning of that Organ. Greater quantities make an imbalance more extreme.

Consider the foods you have eaten recently (either from the list you made from the Action Box on page 33, or just what you have eaten today). Decide which of these foods have which taste. Remember that some foods may have more than one taste:

- How well balanced are the tastes of your food?
- Which taste do you eat the most?
- Which taste do you eat least?

Could you eat a better balance of these tastes? If so, how might you do this?

Indira's diet

Indira is 54 and is married with grown-up children. She came to England from India six years ago and feels settled in London where she lives. She works in her husband's shop during the day. Recently she has become worried about her health. Her doctor has told her that her blood pressure is getting quite high and she has also been getting indigestion and heartburn quite severely. This is what Indira eats on a normal day:

8.00   *Breakfast*: Spicy parathas made from special wheat flour and stuffed with potatoes.

12.30   *Lunch*: Spicy dahl (which is made from lentils) with rice and cooked vegetables.

6.00   *Supper*: Plain chapatis with spicy chicken curry, rice and vegetables. Milk pudding. A glass of water.

Between meals she drinks plain water or a special Indian brew of tea.

Indira's dietary problems

The spicy food in Indira's diet is causing most of her problems. When she was in India this spicy food was a necessary part of the diet – the chilli peppers made her perspire and cooled her down in the strong heat. Now in England she is still eating the same diet but the climate is cold and damp and she doesn't perspire. The spicy food is staying in her system and is causing her Stomach and Liver to overheat. The heat is causing her blood pressure to rise and is also irritating her stomach.

Suggestions for Indira

- **Cut down on the spicy food**. Indira uses large quantities of chilli powder in each meal. She is advised to cut it by half.

- **Cut down on salt**. She uses a lot of salt in her cooking and this is putting a strain on her system, causing her blood pressure to rise.

- **Use less grease in cooking**. A lot of the ingredients of the dahl are cooked in oil and the vegetables are stir-fried.

Indira's basic diet is good. She eats at regular times and has a large amount of grains, beans and vegetables.

25 Find tasty substitutes

If you need to give up or reduce your intake of certain foods it is always best to substitute with an alternative. Here are some suggestions.

Dairy products

Replace with oat or rice milk, or alternatively try almond or quinoa milk. You could also use small amounts of sheep's or goat's cheese, yoghurt or milk.

Orange juice

Dilute apple, pear or grape juice concentrate, or drink mineral water.

Coffee and tea

It may be easiest to change to decaffeinated coffee or tea, although make sure it is carried out by a natural water process. Other alternatives are herb teas or my personal favourite is rooibos (redbush) tea, which is low in caffeine and tannin. There are many coffee substitutes such as 'Caro' or 'Barleycup' but coffee addicts may find these harder to change to as they might be considered a poor substitute for the real thing!

Hot spices

Use milder herbs for flavouring or a smaller amounts of spices. Soya sauce is also a good alternative.

Sugary foods

Use foods with a natural sweetness such as sweet potatoes, parsnips, carrots or peas (not frozen with added sugar!). Alternatively use foods that have been naturally sweetened with apple juice or molasses. Avoid most artificial sweeteners, although a sweetener called Xylitol is an excellent one – it is natural, and good for the teeth as well. Carob is a useful substitute for chocolate (an acquired taste if you're a chocoholic!).

Fatty red meat

Eat more fish (oily fish such as sardines and mackerel is best) and poultry. Eat tofu burgers and sausages, and bean and lentil dishes.

Alcohol

Drink an occasional low-alcohol lager, or alternatively organic wine or beer.

Wheat

Eat rice, oats, rye and products made from other grains (see page 35 for cooking grains). Also eat fresh rye bread or pumpernickel bread. Use wheat-free pasta and other similar products. Eat oat biscuits or rice cakes. Find wheat-free 'bars' for a healthy snack – usually available in health food shops. There is also much gluten-free food (which contains no wheat, oats, rye or barley) in the supermarkets now, and shops often have a 'free from' section where you can buy gluten-free and other allergen-free foods.

Action Box

There are many reasons for cutting out certain foods from your diet. You may try excluding some foods because you are wondering if you are sensitive to them (see page 72). Alternatively you may just want to move to a healthier diet. Whatever the reason, never remove a food from your diet without replacing it with a tasty alternative. If you don't have a substitute you are likely to start craving the food you have given up and go back to it before you have adjusted to the change.

Remember to keep the amount of food you eat in balance when substituting or changing your diet. Food that is healthy in smaller quantities can be unhealthy when taken in larger amounts. For example, a small amount of sweet food is good for you but large amounts weaken your Stomach and Spleen.

26 Eat regular meals

Chinese medicine recommends that we eat three main meals a day with a break of approximately five hours between each meal. So, for example, if we have breakfast at 7.00 a.m., our evening meal will be around 6.00 p.m. A Chinese dietary classic, written over two thousand years ago, the *Lu Shi Chun Qiu*, says 'One is sure to be free from disease if he (or she) keeps regular dining hours.'[35]

Don't miss meals

Consistency is very important, as the Stomach likes regularity. When we eat regularly, we start to feel hungry as we mentally and physically prepare to eat. The result is better spaced-out energy throughout the day. If we miss meals this will deplete our *qi* and imbalance the Stomach and Spleen, which are the main Organs of digestion.

Creating a routine stabilizes our dietary habits. This means that we are less likely to eat convenience foods and we will eat in a way that is good for our health and wellbeing.

Eat breakfast to maintain your energy

Eating breakfast ensures we have energy to last us through the day. Research confirms the importance of eating breakfast. A study of 2,216 teenagers found that those who ate breakfast were more likely to have a lower body mass index (BMI) and have healthier eating habits five years later than those who skip it.

The principal investigator of the project said this study confirmed the importance of helping teenagers to learn to start the day 'right' by eating breakfast: 'Although they may think that skipping breakfast seems like a good way to save on calories, findings suggest the opposite.'[36]

Avoid eating late at night

If we eat late at night our body will not have enough time to digest our food before we go to sleep. Our sleep should nourish us. If we are still digesting food at night, less energy will be available to replenish us and we may wake up feeling tired. Continually eating late can also lead to the nourishing *yin* aspect of our digestion becoming deficient, making it more difficult to settle inside and leading to insomnia or light sleeping. It can also contribute to even more serious illnesses such as diabetes.

Action Box

Create a dietary routine

Each of us needs to create our own personal routine and to consider the times when we eat during the day. It is best that this includes eating three meals a day. Creating a routine stabilizes our dietary habits. This means that we are less likely to eat convenience foods and we will eat in a way that is good for our health and wellbeing.

If you skip breakfast your energy level may drop later in the morning. This can cause cravings for chocolate or other sugary snacks. On the other hand if you are still digesting food at night, less energy will be available to replenish you and you may wake up feeling tired.

Remember the saying: **'Breakfast like a king, lunch like a prince and dine like a pauper.**

27 Eat in the right conditions

As well as eating regularly, we can also strive to eat in conditions that assist our Stomach and Spleen to assimilate our food. This includes resting after eating, chewing our food well, eating until we are 70% full and eating in a calm environment.

Nowadays many people don't find the time to sit down and digest their food properly. Compare this with what Chinese wisdom teaches us about eating.

Chinese people typically take their lunch and then relax and maybe even cat-nap for half an hour afterwards. The cat-nap will allow them to digest their food and prepare for their afternoon activities. This strategy means that they feel ready to accomplish their tasks twice as efficiently as those who have not taken a break (see Secret 57 for more on resting during the day).

Action Box

Eat in the right conditions

Rest after eating. Even if you don't rest for a full half hour after eating take some time to ensure you digest your food before moving on to other activities.

Always sit down to eat and allow some time to digest your meal properly. Preferably find somewhere to eat lunch away from your normal workspace. Don't eat on the run. Take a short rest after eating lunch. This should be no more than half an hour but will prepare you for the afternoon's activities.

Eat only until you're 70% full. A famous Chinese medicine doctor, Ao Ying, says: 'man should endure 30 per cent hunger and up to 70 per cent fullness.'[37] Chinese medicine says that eating until we are full up and bloated will strain the Stomach and Spleen *qi*. Another famous Chinese text, *Nei Jing* states: 'Overeating impairs the Intestines and the Stomach' (see page 136 for more on 'the 70%' rule).

Don't eat a meal while you're still digesting a previous meal. This can lead to the contents of your Stomach stagnating and can cause indigestion.

Chew your food well. This helps the digestive juices to break down your food. It's also better to talk *between* mouthfuls rather than while you are actually chewing your food.

Eat in a calm environment. If possible, it is better not to eat while you're angry or unhappy as it is more difficult to digest food in these circumstances. It is also better to avoid eating while watching television, reading, discussing emotional issues or doing anything that takes your mind away from your food.

Avoid eating too much cold food. The body needs heat in order to digest food. Cold food slows down our metabolism.

Many of us may remember that our grandparents also took this time to relax. After lunch, people would often have half-an-hour's rest before going back to work again. It is now common for people to eat their food rapidly and on the run and take a very short lunch-break instead of sitting down to eat properly. Often people take their meals while they are stressed or involved in other activities such as watching television, reading a book, sitting at their computer or making business deals.

Action Box

A summary of the ways you can balance your lifestyle in relation to your dietary habits:

- Eat regularly.

- Avoiding eating late at night.

- Allow time for digestion.

- Eat only until you're 70% full.

- Don't eat a meal while you're still digesting a previous meal.

- Eat three meals a day including breakfast.

- Chew your food well.

- Always sit down to eat and allow some time to digest your meal properly.

- Eat in a calm environment.

- Avoid eating too much cold food.

Check how many of the above you achieve regularly and habitually. Then pick out one area you would like to change and think about how you might change it. Decide when and how you are going to put that into practice.

28 Try sprouting – nutritious food from tiny seedlings

Chinese people often use mung bean sprouts in their stir-fries or as a side dish. Sprouted beans, grains or seeds are an inexpensive way to eat fresh and nourishing food. Bean sprouts are packed full of vitamins, minerals, antioxidants and anti-ageing constituents and are probably one of the most nutritious foods available.

It is easy to sprout seedlings. Once you have found a suitable container and high-quality seeds (always use organic) there is very little for you to do. As long as you rinse them twice a day they will easily grow and can be harvested as a tasty dish after a few days.

Try sprouting these beans and grains:

- **Alfalfa:** an easy seed to sprout and a good one to start with. It's very tasty, great in a sandwiches and will be ready to eat in 5–7 days.

- **Mung beans:** very tasty and sweet and can be harvested after about 5 days. Don't leave them much longer as they can grow too long and then taste bitter.

- **Aduki beans:** these have a good taste and take about 5 days to grow.

- **Lentils:** these can be eaten fresh or steamed. They are easy to grow and ready in 5 days.

- **Sunflower seeds:** these have a sweet nutty taste if eaten after 2 days. Don't leave for too long as they can start to taste bitter and easily go mouldy.

You can also try sprouting chickpeas, barley, oat groats, kamut wheat – or experiment with many other grains, beans or seeds.

Many containers can be used for sprouting. One of the most common is a jar covered in muslin as the lid. Alternatively use a sprouting tray. Many styles of tiered sprouting trays are now on sale and these are clean and simple to use.

Seeds will not germinate if they are:

- of poor quality

- placed too close together

- not kept watered

- not kept at the right temperature (ideally 18–22 °C).

Action Box

Sprouting seeds

- Place a tablespoon of the seeds or beans in the container. Bear in mind that sprouting increases the volume of the seeds by 6–8 times so a small amount will go a long way.
- Cover with water and soak for approximately 8 hours, then drain away the water.
- Rinse the sprouts twice a day by pouring water through the container. Do not leave them immersed in water as this will cause them to rot. If they are not rinsed through they will dry out and die.

Once they have sprouted, use in a stir-fry or as a side dish or steamed.
If you don't wish to use the bean sprouts immediately store them in a cool dark place (a fridge is good), where they will usually keep for a week.

29 Know how and when to drink fluids

Chinese medicine suggests that we sip drinks between meals rather than at mealtimes. There is a saying that we should 'chew our drink and drink our food'.

If we 'chew' our drinks we will only take them in small amounts, allowing them to be thoroughly 'rotted and ripened'. Drinking vast amounts of fluid along with our food tends to flood the Stomach and Spleen and washes our food down. This gives our digestion more work to do. We can also 'drink' our food until it becomes like fluid. This stimulates saliva and will aid the first stage of digestion, which is in the mouth.

It is best to also avoid caffeinated drinks, like tea and coffee and colas, as they are over-stimulating. I have seen many patients complaining of insomnia, anxiety and heart palpitations who have cured their symptoms just by cutting down their excessive amounts of caffeinated drinks.

It is best to drink warm water (not ice cold) or herb teas or, of course, China's favourite drink, green tea (see Secret 30).

It is also best not to drink anything that is too rich such as juices like orange juice (see page 56).

Action Box

Consider all the fluids you usually drink in a day (either from the list you made from the Action Box on page 33, or just what you have drunk yesterday or today).

- How much of the drink was extremely caffeinated?
- What was your alcohol intake?
- What percentage of your fluid intake was hot or what percentage was cold?
- Did you sip your drinks between meals or take them with meals?
- How much water did you drink?

Consider how balanced you think this was and if it would be beneficial to change it.

30 Drink green tea or other healthy drinks

The Book of Tea by Lu Yu was written as early as the Tang dynasty (618–905). It describes the health benefits of green tea. Green tea is the most widely consumed drink in the world after water and has long been known by the Chinese to have a extensive list of health benefits. These have been borne out by more recent research.

Some of the effects of green tea are quite astounding. Green tea contains many powerful antioxidants, vitamins (especially A, C and E) and minerals (especially selenium). It is known to have cancer fighting effects, to combat heart disease, to fight many bacteria, to inhibit the effect of viruses, to aid weight loss, stimulate the immune system, lower cholesterol and prevent ageing.[38] Many of the diseases of the 21st century could be prevented by taking green tea along with a healthy diet.

Although green tea, like black tea and coffee, does contain caffeine it is in much smaller quantities. Depending on how it is brewed, fresh coffee contains 80–115 mg of caffeine and black tea approximately 40. In comparison green tea, brewed for three minutes, contains only 15 mg. It would take four cups of the strongest green tea to equal one cup of the weakest brewed coffee.[39]

The Chinese tend to sip tea between meals when they are resting and not at mealtimes. They would also suggest not drinking it before bed. Besides having a slightly diuretic quality it is also quite stimulating. It can 'refresh the brain and get rid of fatigue'.[40] These are useful effects during the day but do not encourage a long, deep sleep.

Action Box

Green tea can be an acquired taste – and everyone has their own drinking preferences. Consider which drinks you find tasty and be aware of how healthy they are. If you drink a lot of tea, coffee, colas and other caffeinated drinks, be aware of their potential long-term negative effect on your health. Women take longer to detoxify and recover from their stimulating effects.[41] Cutting back on caffeine has been shown to have a marked reduction in PMT symptoms including breast tenderness, irritability and other symptoms such as cramps, bloating and nausea.[42] Drinks high in caffeine create an increased risk of osteoporosis,[43] hot flushes in menopause[44] and heart attacks[45] and elevate stress levels.[46]

31 Be alert for food sensitivities

Food sensitivities are very common these days and seem to arise from imbalances in our modern-day diets and lifestyles. If we relax and 'listen' to our bodies we will become increasingly aware of which foods enhance our health and which make us less healthy. There are a number of ways that might help us to notice how we are reacting.

Listen to your body

If we tune into our bodies for a few minutes after eating we might notice certain responses that let us know that our body is sensitive to a particular food. Common responses are:

- feeling bloated after eating
- a feeling of phlegm arising in the throat or chest
- headaches
- indigestion
- belching and wind
- discomfort in the stomach area
- general lethargy
- heaviness.

These are just a few of many possible responses. It can be important to spend time noticing the different effects of certain foods.

Food cravings

Any extreme craving or dislike of a food may indicate that we are sensitive to it. It's ironic that the foods we crave are often the ones that have the most negative effect on our health. If you notice a craving for a specific food it may initially take a great deal of motivation to eliminate that food from your diet. It's probably best to stop eating the 'offending' food for just a few weeks and to see what difference it makes to your health. If by then you are feeling better you may be motivated to cut it out completely. It won't be long before the craving disappears and is replaced by a feeling of relief that you've eliminated a food that is not beneficial to your health.

'Suspect' food

Sometimes we don't have cravings or responses to eating certain foods but still wonder if our symptoms are due to our diet. After reading this chapter, for example, you might decide you need fewer phlegm and damp-forming foods, or need to add more vegetables or meat to your diet. In this case, make the alteration and then note if your health improves over a period of three or four weeks. This will signal if the change has been a positive one.

Remember that foods come in groups – for example, dairy produce covers a wide range of foods including cheese, butter and cream – and that there are a large number of foods with eggs or sugar in them.

Food substitution

We mentioned earlier how important it is to substitute foods when changing our diets rather than just cutting them out (see page 61). You might like to prepare in advance when planning to eliminate foods from your diet and find tasty substitutes beforehand. Make use of the wide variety of foods available in supermarkets and whole or health food shops. If we don't substitute it may be far more difficult to make the changes we require. If we search out substitutes we enjoy, the adjustments become easy.

Action Box

Some signs and symptoms are triggered by an intolerance or sensitivity to certain foods or food additives. If you suspect that you are sensitive to one or more foods, try the following:

- Remove one or more of the suspect foods from your diet completely for a few weeks.
- Notice if the symptom recedes during this time.
- If the symptom recedes, cut out the food(s) for a longer period and note whether the symptom continues to abate.

Food sensitivities can occur if we eat an excessive amount of one type of food over long periods, or if at an early age we were given food that our digestive system was not mature enough to digest. If we crave one particular food this may be a sign that we are sensitive to it. Sadly, we may need to give up the very food we most enjoy in order to overcome the symptoms of intolerance.

Hannah's diet

Hannah is 19 and works in an office from 9 a.m. to 5 p.m. She has problems with her weight and finds it fluctuates a lot. She has recently started feeling bloated after her meals. She also finds she gets spots on her face, especially before her period and she is also often constipated. This is what she eats on a normal day:

8.00   Cup of coffee. Leaves for work having skipped breakfast.
10.00   Chocolate bar.
1.00   Sandwich – either cheese or egg salad, a packet of crisps and an apple.
3.00   Biscuit.
5.00   Leaves work. May have a chocolate biscuit or two when she gets home.
6.30   Heats up a pre-cooked meal from the supermarket with vegetables.

Coffee and tea throughout the day sweetened with an artificial sweetener.

Hannah's dietary problems

Hannah's main problem is a weak Spleen. The Spleen is responsible for transporting food and drink in the body. Her current diet is not nourishing her Spleen and she is eating excessively sweet-tasting food which is further weakening her Spleen. The Spleen deficiency is making her bloat, is causing her intestines to become sluggish and is giving her spots.

Suggestions for Hannah

Hannah is advised to add more nourishing food to her diet:

- **Take the time to eat a nourishing breakfast.** She may have to get up slightly earlier to do this but a warming bowl of porridge will set her up for the day. Her blood sugar has probably been dropping in the mid-morning, causing her to crave chocolate, and a good breakfast will stop this happening.

- **Substitute healthier snacks.** If she finds it difficult to cut out the chocolate she can do it gradually. Carob can substitute for chocolate until she loses the addiction or she could try snacks sweetened with apple juice or molasses.

- **Eat a hot meal at lunchtime.** Take a hot nourishing soup. A vegetable soup made the night before will fill her up. This can be eaten with a wholemeal roll or rice cakes.

- **Eat more fruit, vegetables and grains.** She could put fruit on her porridge. She already gets vegetables in the evening and this is good. Avoiding the pre-cooked meals and making rice dishes or wholemeal pasta would be a healthier choice for the evening.

- **Substitute alternative drinks for tea and coffee.** Artificial sweeteners encourage her taste for sweet food. Occasional tea and coffee is fine but she needs to drink far less of it. She can start with naturally caffeine-free tea such as rooibos and coffee substitutes.

These are a lot of changes for Hannah to make so she might choose to do them gradually. She could start with the porridge, hot soup and healthy evening meal. As she notices the difference to her health she might feel inspired to make more changes.

If you are ill it is always best to get the advice of a doctor or a practitioner of Chinese medicine rather than trying to cure yourself by diet alone.

4 Secrets to Balance Our Emotions

Our emotions and our health

Our emotions reflect the movements of our *qi*. If our *qi* is flowing smoothly our emotions are expressed in a balanced way. When we respond negatively to a situation, we tighten up inside, causing our *qi* to become blocked or to travel in the wrong direction. The famous Chinese medical textbook, the *Nei Jing* says: 'Anger makes *qi* rise, joy slows down *qi*, sadness dissolves *qi*, fear makes *qi* descend . . . shock scatters *qi* . . . worry knots *qi*.'[1]

Chinese medicine recognizes that anger, fear, joy, grief, shock, worry and sadness are all emotions that can affect our health. The emotions are called the 'internal causes' of disease because we generate them from inside ourselves. In contrast, weather conditions like heat, cold or damp are called 'external causes' of disease. 'Lifestyle causes' such as diet, exercise or overwork are referred to as 'not internal and not external'.

Although Chinese medicine names only seven emotions as internal causes, these seven include all other emotions, as listed below.

- **Anger:** frustration, depression, resentment, irritation, bitterness, rage, wrath, ire.

- **Fear:** fright, terror, anxiety, dread, panic, trepidation, apprehension, horror, foreboding.

- **Grief:** loss, emptiness, resignation, longing, regret, remorse, mourning, feeling bereft.

- **Over-joyousness:** excitement, elation, euphoria, exhilaration, excessive enthusiasm, mania.

- **Sadness:** misery, unhappiness, despair, gloom, sorrow, flatness, melancholy, downhearted.

- **Worry:** obsession, over-thinking, fixation, fretfulness, angst, over-concern, insecurity.

- **Shock:** fright, alarm, agitation, distress, shaken up, stirred up, startled, disquiet.

It is natural for us to experience different emotions according to our circumstances. For instance:

- Fear protects us from danger.

- Anger helps us to assert our rights.

- Grief manifests when we lose someone or something.

- Joy arises when we feel pleasure.

- Worry occurs when we feel unsupported.

Once the situation that has aroused our emotion has subsided we usually recover and let it go. There are other circumstances, however, when we don't recover. Then these emotions can negatively affect our health.

In this chapter we discuss some ways of dealing with 'stuck' emotions so that they don't injure our health. I have taken these suggestions from many sources. Some are modern ways of dealing with emotions, others are older and derived directly from Chinese culture. All are written in the 'spirit' of Chinese medicine and the understanding that resolving emotional problems can prevent disease.

32 Emotions are a key to good health

When emotions cause disease

All emotions are normal and appropriate under certain circumstances. They only tend to cause disease when they are prolonged, intense, not expressed or not acknowledged.

The timing of emotional traumas

Emotional traumas can start in childhood – a time when we have no means of protecting ourselves. As children we rely on our parents to love, protect and nurture us, as well as to show us right from wrong and teach us boundaries. Not many of us would say that we had a perfect childhood, but what devastates one child may have little or no effect on another. Children may be disturbed by a variety of events, such as being bullied at school, being scared of exams, moving home, losing friends, or parents quarrelling.

Traumas that take place later in life can also have a huge impact but don't usually go quite as deep as childhood events. The death of a loved one or the break up of a relationship, for example, is a shattering ordeal. These events are difficult to deal with but usually heal over time, if we allow them to and get the support we need.

Short-lived or long term?

Some emotions are more short term than others. Feeling angry with your spouse for being late to a meal is one thing. Long-term, bottled-up anger following continual mental or physical abuse is very different. The best thing is to deal with emotional traumas in the present, then you will have fewer stuck emotions in the future. If you can clear anger out of your system you won't bottle up more potential ill-health in the future.

How we deal with our emotions

Each individual has a different attitude to the traumatic life events they have gone through. Some people feel that they can never get over the upsets of the past. Others feel that they can learn from their problems and become better people for it.

A counsellor I know works with people who are in severe distress. In her experience some people who have had appalling difficulties can manage to use and learn from them, while others seem to go round and round, digging a deeper and deeper hole, unable to get out.

So what is it that enables one person to deal with their emotional difficulties while another is unable to? The answer is complex. A healthy childhood involves small to medium frustrations from which the child can learn. The depth and intensity of a trauma, the timing of the difficulties and the length of time they continue are relevant to whether we get through them or whether they cause problems later.

Physical illness and its emotional component

It has been said that approximately 90% of all illness has an emotional component. In spite of this some people can be worried about having illnesses labelled as 'psychosomatic'. The word psychosomatic has negative connotations and we may think that this means our symptoms aren't real or are 'inferior' to physical ones. In this case we might deny that our problems are affecting us.

You may imagine that you can withstand all difficulties in life and your health will remain unscathed. This denial may also mean that you don't ask for help and don't accept help when it is offered. You may also keep your feelings locked inside, and your body has to deal with the resulting blockage or depletion caused by the unresolved emotions. This denial can manifest as illness later on.

A patient recently told me that after a marriage break-up his whole body deteriorated. His bowels became irregular and he had discomfort in his chest and stomach all the time. Later he was diagnosed as having both asthma and irritable bowel syndrome. Inside he knew that he had never got over the anger and distress. At the time of the break-up he had tensed up inside, pretending he was coping. This caused his *qi* to stop flowing smoothly. The root of his problem had been unresolved emotions. Acupuncture treatment, which helped to move his *qi*, as well as learning to deal with his emotions, were the first steps to regaining his health.

> ### Action Box
>
> One important factor in the face of difficulties is acceptance. Accepting that problems are there and how they affect us can enable us to keep them in perspective. It may stop us from becoming overwhelmed by them and prevent us from suppressing or denying them. We may then be able to let them go rather than letting them becoming prolonged, intense or unacknowledged – which can lead to ill-health.

Common stresses through stages in our lives

Infancy (0–5)
Lack of food; lack of warm environment; lack of emotional warmth and stimulation; lack of ability to get emotional needs met; lack of or too many physical boundaries; sibling rivalries; separating from parents as we grow older.

Childhood (5–12)
Starting school; making friends; learning difficulties; sibling rivalry; bullying; moving home; parents divorcing; keeping up with schoolwork; too much television, too many computer games.

Teenage years (13–19)
Starting relationships with same or opposite sex; making friends; concern about appearance; fear of failing exams; difficulty choosing a career; becoming independent from parents; experimenting with drugs and/or alcohol; finding work; leaving home.

Adulthood (20–40)

Finding a partner; building a home; starting a family; finding and settling in a career; financial worries and debts; competitive work situation; difficult boss; difficulties with colleagues; relationship problems; divorce.

Late adulthood (40–60)

Redundancy; lack of promotion; keeping up with changes in technology at work; caring for ageing parents; family illness; death of relatives and friends; advancing age; declining health; possible divorce.

Retirement (60+)

Lack of feeling valued; death of loved ones; failing health; advancing age; failing eyesight, hearing, memory, etc.; loss of income; loss of ability to care for self; difficulty maintaining independence.

33 Anger makes *qi* rise

Much research has been carried out into the effect of anger on our health. One study conducted at universities in Miami and California involved 27 people. Two-thirds were suffering from heart disease and one-third were not. The subjects were tested while they were exercising and also while undergoing psychological stressors. The psychological stressors included making a speech, doing mental arithmetic and recalling an event that made them angry. The study found that everyone's heart was more affected by situations that made them angry than by exercise or any of the other psychological stressors.[2]

Chinese medicine teaches us that the organs have 'functions' beyond the characteristics defined by Western medicine. Different emotions affect these functions in the different organs. Anger will affect the functions connected to the Liver. Interestingly, one Liver function is to allow the *qi* to flow smoothly and easily throughout the body. If the *qi* flow is smooth then we are relaxed. When we are angry or tense the *qi* can become constricted. Many of the symptoms of premenstrual tension are due to this lack of free-flowing *qi*. Other symptoms include tension, bloating, swollen breasts and mood swings.

One patient became ill because of frustration at work. She went into a human resources job thinking that she would help people but instead found she was making people redundant! Not surprisingly she found it distressing and frustrating to see people suffering but kept the feelings inside. As a result she had premenstrual tension, mood swings and, in the end, a benign tumour on her spine. That was the real warning sign and she changed her job.

The increasing pace of life results in more tension and we may feel under pressure. We need to find better ways of dealing with the diseases that result from stress. Treating only the symptoms of stress is not enough. Chinese medicine and all holistic therapies teach that dealing with the underlying cause is the only way truly to tackle ill-health. Unexpressed anger is probably one of the most common causes of ill-health in modern-day society.

Should we express our anger or suppress it? People often think that these are the only two options, but there are other ways of dealing with anger. For example, we can realize that we are in control. When we get angry we often think that someone has done something to us and 'made' us angry. Although we may feel like a helpless victim, this is unlikely to be the case. If you frequently feel like a helpless victim, however, it may be a signal that you need to discover more options.

We can look at the thoughts behind our anger – are we assuming that someone is purposely upsetting us? For example, we may think to ourselves: 'If she cared about me she wouldn't leave that mess' or 'If he respected me he would stop saying those things.' People are not always aware of the effect of their actions and even if they are they may find it difficult to change them.

We can also consider whether our situation is really important enough to get angry about. Ask yourself, will this make a difference to my life in an hour, a week or a year?

Other signs and symptoms that result from *qi* rising upwards or not flowing smoothly include eye problems, headaches and digestive complaints such as sour regurgitation or belching. Also dizziness, muscle tension, spasms, a tight chest, moodiness or any symptom (including pain) that comes and goes, moves around or changes in intensity.

Action Box

Making an anger inventory

Everybody gets angry sometimes and it may be important to do so when we wish to assert ourselves or make changes. If we never show anger at all, or we become angry and uptight at the slightest provocation, then both of these may injure our health. The following questions will help you to assess whether your feelings of anger are occasional or chronic, and if they are chronic if they are likely to be affecting your health.

- What kinds of situations make you angry?
- Where do you feel it in your body?
- How often do you become angry in a day?
- When you get angry how do you express it?
- Are you able to sort frustrations out or do you hold on to them and fume for days?
- Do you have any of the signs and symptoms listed in the section above?

If you realize that you are getting angry every day without resolving the feelings, this may be a signal that you need to do more to deal with it. Many of the exercises in this book will help you to deal with emotions including anger. Secrets 8, 39, 40, 41, 42, 43, 46, 47, 57 and 65 may be especially helpful.

---

34 Fear makes *qi* descend and worry knots the *qi*

When we feel angry we are responding to something from either the past or the present. In contrast, fear, anxiety and worry are linked to the future. Often the events we anticipate don't materialize. If you are a persistent worrier, even knowing that you have wasted time feeling highly stressed for no good reason doesn't help you to stop.

Worry and anxiety often affect the Stomach and other digestive functions, as one of my patients discovered. She told me that worrying had a direct effect on her health. Even if it was only a slight worry it all went straight to her guts. 'When I've got to get a lot done my guts will tighten up.' She noticed that when she was not worried she would be calm and settled and her health was much better.

Research carried out at Yale University into the effects of stress found that it had a significant impact on many gastro-intestinal disorders, and on other diseases such as asthma, diabetes, heart problems, some forms of rheumatoid arthritis, many cancers and even our propensity to get colds. We saw in Chapter 3 that diet plays an important role in our health – stress has been found to be an important factor too.[3]

Other signs and symptoms might include urinary problems, incontinence, poor energy or lethargy, swollen legs, a bloated abdomen, digestive problems such as indigestion and discomfort in the stomach area, loose stools, prolapsed organs or weak limbs.

Action Box

Dealing with fear, anxiety and worry

Fear, anxiety and worry do have a positive as well as a negative side. Fear protects us from danger. It alerts us to threats and prepares us to take action in dangerous situations. Worry occurs when a need for support arises. It enables us to plan to deal with difficult situations.

If we are continually fearful, anxious or worried we will contract against non-existent threats or become 'knotted up' when going over and over our concerns. If these feelings are more extreme than is warranted by the real danger or concern, then they may be out of balance.

These questions will help you to assess whether you are occasionally fearful, anxious or worried, or if these are feelings you experience on a daily basis and could therefore be affecting your health:

- What kinds of situations make you fearful, anxious or worried?
- Where in your body do you feel these feelings?

- How often do you become fearful, anxious or worried in a day?
- When you have these feelings how do you deal with them?
- Do you go over and over your concerns and fears for days or can you let go of them?
- Do you have any of the signs and symptoms listed in the section above?

If you know your fear, anxiety or worries are affecting your daily life it may be an important signal that these emotions need to be dealt with. Many of the exercises in this book can help you to deal with your feelings. Secrets 8, 9, 37, 39, 40, 44, 46, 47 and 59 may be especially helpful.

35 Grief and sadness dissolve *qi*

In 1975, 26 bereaved spouses were brave enough to take part in a study into the effect of stress on the immune system. They were tested two weeks after their bereavement and again six weeks later. A 'control' group made up of 26 people who had not been bereaved within the previous two years was also tested. The study showed clearly that the immune system of those who were recently bereaved was severely depressed while that of the control group remained normal. The 26 bereaved spouses were more prone to illness during this extremely stressful period.[4]

Infections are not the only problems to follow bereavement. The resulting suppressed immune system can cause cancer, arthritis, intestinal problems and many other conditions.

The normal stages we experience when we are going through the grieving process are:[5]

- Denial – it can't be happening.

- Anger – why me? It's not fair.

- Bargaining – trying to reverse the loss by offering exchanges.

- Depression – feeling of intense sadness.

- Acceptance – it's going to be OK.

Not all these stages necessarily occur when we experience a loss, and they can appear in any order. Once we are through this grieving process we can move on. If we do not move on, and stay grieving, we can injure our long-term health.

Fortunately, counselling is now widely available for those who have undergone bereavement or other shock. The feelings could otherwise stay inside and cause illness later on in life.

Other signs and symptoms resulting from our *qi* being dissolved and becoming depleted include shortness of breath, a weak voice, dislike of speaking, easily catching colds, panic attacks, poor concentration, listlessness or general weakness, daytime sweating or palpitations.

Action Box

Responding to grief and sadness

We think of grief occurring when someone close to us dies, but loss can take many other forms. We may feel grief when a relationship ends, or even when we lose something that is of value to us, such as a piece of jewellery or an article of clothing. Or we may feel loss if a dream or something we might like to happen or have done never manifests.

Some people are grieving when there is no obvious loss or they may be unable to move on from a loss that has occurred many years before. We know we feel grief and sadness if we continually have an empty feeling inside.

The questions below will help you to assess your feelings of grief or sadness and whether or not you are moving on from them:

- Do you regularly feel empty or sad?
- If you have these feelings, how do you deal with them?
- What kinds of situations make you sad or bring on feelings of grief?

- Where in your body do you feel grief and sadness?
- Do you have any of the signs and symptoms listed in the above section?

If you have had a recent bereavement then your grief may be a part of a natural healing process and it needs to be expressed. Or you may recognize that grief and sadness are affecting you and you are not dealing with these feelings. In this case you may find many of the tips in this and other chapters useful. Secrets 8, 40, 42, 43, 44, 47 and 55 may be especially helpful.

36 Joy slows *qi* down

Although good feelings can be beneficial to our health, joy can also be a cause of disease. We might wonder how joy could have any negative effects but Chinese medicine understands that any extreme emotion can cause illness. 'Joy' is imbalanced when it manifests as overexcitement, euphoria and agitation. If we experience sudden and overwhelming feelings of joy we can be left wide open. We may temporarily feel wonderful but as a result our resistance to disease is lowered and we often feel low afterwards. If that dream of winning the lottery came true it might not be so good for our health!

It is interesting to note that a prayer by St Augustine says: 'Tend thy sick ones, O Lord Christ; rest thy weary ones; bless thy dying ones; soothe thy suffering ones; shield thy joyous ones; and all for thy love's sake.'[6]

An extreme form of joy can occur in manic behaviour. Someone may remain excessively joyful and overactive for long periods of time, but eventually they can burn themselves out. The other side of this 'joy' is unhappiness.

It is possible to laugh and show joy to the world when inside you are deeply unhappy. An acupuncture student I know always seems bright and cheerful and people often remark on it. When learning about the Heart and its connection to joy she tried to think of past situations when she had felt joyful. She was shocked to realize that in spite of her cheerfulness she could not remember a single time when she had experienced being truly joyful. Underneath her external cheerfulness she realized that she felt quite unhappy.

Signs and symptoms resulting from your *qi* being slowed down or unsettled include poor concentration, confusion, stuffiness or pain in the heart region, mania, excessive restlessness or insomnia.

Action Box

Exploring agitated feelings

We are all likely to feel unsettled and agitated at certain times. But continual agitation or overexcitement is not healthy and it may be a sign that you're overdoing things and 'running on empty'.

The following questions will help you to assess your unsettled feelings and whether they are affecting your health:

- Do you often feel 'up' or elated, and unable to settle?
- Are you ever able to be settled and peaceful with yourself?
- If you feel unsettled, where in your body do you feel it?
- Do you have any of the signs and symptoms listed above?

If you think you are overexcited or agitated look through the exercises in the rest of this chapter, find one that suits you and try it for a month. Secrets 39, 40, 42, 43, 47, 51, 57, 58 and 59 may be especially useful.

---

37 Take pleasure from the world

During the Ming dynasty (1368–1644), a Chinese scholar, Wang Xunan, suggested that we can stay contented by 'taking pleasure from the world', and this in turn can enable us to have a long and happy life.[7] We can take pleasure in many simple things, such as reading a book, walking in the countryside, feeling a warm breeze, admiring beautiful paintings, talking to a friend, listening to music or looking at beautiful flowers. These are all opportunities to appreciate life.

Action Box

One way to help you to take pleasure in life, on a daily basis, is to keep a journal. In this journal write down three things each day in answer to the following questions.

In the morning on waking, ask yourself:

- What do I appreciate in my life at present?
- What am I enjoying about my life at present?

In the evening you can then ask yourself:

- What have I learnt from today?
- What have I given out today?

By doing this regularly you will soon start to see life from another point of view.

Writing a journal can bring many benefits. One patient told me that writing kept her calm when disasters seemed about to strike. Another said a journal kept her difficulties in perspective.

The things we note down and appreciate can be exceptional or more mundane. We may be grateful to someone who listens to us or just be pleased that we've cooked a decent supper. We might be grateful for intangible things such as having clarity of mind or that a friend wants our help. We might appreciate more concrete things – a bargain jumper bought in the sales or good film that made us laugh.

There's always something we can take pleasure from even when things are really tough. One patient who described herself as chronically discontented kept an appreciation journal for over a year. She told me she'd learnt three things:

- Our difficulties always pass.

- Most people have a good heart.

- It's usually the small things that bring her *real* pleasure.

As a result she has become more satisfied and comfortable with her day-to-day life.

38 Know the importance of humour

Two well-known and much quoted Chinese proverbs state: 'A person should laugh three times a day to live longer,' and: 'A good laugh makes you ten years younger, while worry turns the hair grey.' We may once have regarded these as light-hearted sayings. Research has shown, however, that laughing and keeping positive really are the secrets of good health.

Research carried out at the State University of New York found that laughter increased the levels of an antibody called 'immunoglobulin A', which is found in the lining of the nose and helps the body to fight illnesses. People with fewer antibodies were more prone to colds and other infections. The researchers asked 72 men to fill in a form every evening for 12 weeks, describing how their day had been. Each man also took daily a mucus sample that was analysed for antibody levels. The research found that the level of antibodies was higher on the days where the men had laughed a lot or good things had happened, while on bad days the antibody level was lower.[8]

Other research has found that people who are optimistic are likely to be healthier later on in their life than those who are pessimistic. One study began in the 1940s. Ninety-nine healthy and successful graduates from Harvard University filled out questionnaires that determined their level of optimism or pessimism. They then completed questionnaires each year and were examined by a physician every five years until the age of 60.

Although all graduates were healthy when they left Harvard, the results showed that pessimism in early adulthood is a risk factor for ill-health in middle and late adulthood. Of the 99, 13 had died before the age of 60. Those who were more optimistic remained in better health and were at their healthiest between 40 and 45. Stunningly, there was a less than 1 in 1,000 chance that these results were random – not even the statistical link between lung cancer and smoking is as strong as that![9]

We can see the power of a positive state of mind from the examples above. What is being proved in the West has been known in Chinese culture for thousands of years.

Action Box

During the Ming dynasty Shi Tianji, a Chinese scholar, wrote about the 'Six Always' for maintaining a calm and cheerful state of mind.[10] He recommended that we develop an attitude of looking on the 'bright side of life':

- **Always remain peaceful in mind** – the fewer desires or hopes for personal gain we have, the more peaceful we will become.
- **Always be kind-hearted** – this will help us to gain pleasure from helping other people. If we always think about how others will benefit from what we do then we will have a tranquil mind and a clear conscience.
- **Always uphold justice** – if we hold fast to our integrity in all matters we will be clear about what is right or wrong for us.
- **Always be cheerful** – have a good laugh whenever possible.
- **Always be pleasant** – if we are amiable when dealing with others we will bring happiness to them and ourselves.
- **Always be contented** – although we can't avoid adversity we can strive to remain cheerful when there are troubles.

To carry out all these suggestions throughout our lives would be impossible. Nevertheless, they are a good example of what you might strive towards in order to live happily.

39 Gain perspective on your emotions

The Chinese oracle *I Ching* or *Book of Changes* is around 4,000 years old. It contains some wise words:

Difficulties and obstructions throw a man back on himself. While the inferior man seeks to put the blame on other persons, bewailing his fate, the superior man seeks the error within himself and through this introspection the external obstacle becomes for him an occasion for inner enrichment and education.[11]

An important factor in helping us to deal with our emotional reactions is the ability temporarily to separate ourselves from what we are experiencing. This distance allows us to understand our feelings better. Often we can then learn from what we have experienced and move on.

Action Box

This exercise is especially helpful if you are having difficulty dealing with other people. It will literally enable you to find a new perspective on your situation:

- Find a quiet space where you can relax.
- Think about the situation you are having difficulty with and imagine that you are going through it again. See what you saw when it was happening, hear what you heard and feel any emotions involved. Especially see the other person and notice their breathing, posture, facial expression, gestures and voice tone.
- Now imagine you are looking at the situation from the point of view of a neutral observer. Play an imaginary film of what is happening. Notice from your objective position both what the other person is saying and doing and how you are responding. Observe how both you and the other person trigger each other's reactions. Gently ask yourself, what is the truth of this situation?
- Now see things from the perspective of the other person. Imagine you are that person and can feel as they feel. Gently ask yourself, how does this person experience me?
- You have now considered all positions. Go back to your original feelings and notice if you feel differently about them. You may have found new ways of dealing with the situation.

When we are in conflict it can be easy to look at things only from our own point of view. Our own viewpoint is called 'first position'. In this position, we might blame others for any problems. The viewpoint of the person we are with (and may be in conflict with) is second position. We will find it very hard to see things from the other person's perspective until we have seen the whole situation. We need to look at the circumstances from a distance and this is called the third position, also sometimes known as the position of the 'wise observer'. It is often from this position that we can get in touch with the truth of a situation and find useful ways of dealing with it.[12]

I have taught this exercise many times. One colleague told me that when she gets wound up she now stops herself and looks at the situation from a distance. As a result things don't tick away inside her any more: she used to be like a time bomb waiting to explode. Now she feels able to let go of things – she can see the situation in perspective. She only needed to practise this once or twice before finding it easy to do.

40 Become present to your bodily 'felt sense'

'Focusing' is a method that was devised in the 1960s by a professor from the University of Chicago called Eugene Gendlin. It recognizes, as Chinese medicine does, that difficulties show up in our bodies. With practice it enables us to become *present* to our internal state, rather than avoid, suppress, deny or become overwhelmed by it. When we Focus we find a bodily sense of what is going on and in time this process allows our issues to shift and resolve themselves from the inside.

The importance of checking inside ourselves

Gendlin and his colleagues studied thousands of tapes of therapy sessions in order to discover why some therapy sessions worked and others didn't. Some sessions used classical therapy and others used newer therapies.

As they listened they realized that people didn't change because of the *type* of therapy they were having but because of something they were doing internally. As they went through the therapy they were checking inside themselves for the 'rightness' of what they were doing.

For those who noticed what was happening inside themselves therapy was successful *no matter what style of therapy they did*. For those who didn't check inside it was not as successful. Gendlin developed the Focusing approach in order to teach people how to check on their inner bodily feelings.[13]

When Focusing can be used

You can use Focusing in many situations when you feel uncomfortable inside, such as:

- When uncomfortable thoughts and/or feelings keep going round and round your head.

- If you feel confused about something.

- If you don't know (but want to know) what you feel about something.

- When you're feeling down on yourself.

- If you are just interested in what's going on inside yourself.

How to Focus[14]

Step 1. Find what wants your attention

- Find a quiet, comfortable space.

- Scan through your body, paying attention to how you feel inside. Notice the support of what you're sitting on. Become aware of where your body already feels good or where it feels less clear.

- Notice any feelings of discomfort or thoughts that are nagging you. You might find that there are a number of different feelings inside, for example, a sense of discomfort about an interaction with a colleague at work, a vague ache in your lower abdomen, a slight feeling of sadness in your chest.

- Get a sense of the one thing that most wants your attention. Check inside for a feeling that this is the right one.

Step 2. Get a bodily 'felt sense' of the whole problem

- Do not enter into what you are focusing on as much as get a whole sense of it. Become present to it. Being present is similar to what is called the third position in the previous exercise. It is a neutral and compassionate state that is non-judgemental and accepting. It is important not to become too merged or too distant from the issue you are focusing on.

- The bodily sense (called a 'felt sense') usually starts as a holistic, rather fuzzy and unclear sense of the whole thing. Sit *with* this felt sense, allowing it to form and letting it be there. Patience is needed here. Staying present may take practice.

Step 3. Symbolizing

- Once you are sitting with this unclear felt sense, you might allow a symbol to emerge. The symbol can be a word, a phrase, a picture or a gesture and it will arise from within the felt sense. This may take some time.

Step 4. Resonating

- Once a symbol has arisen, notice how the felt sense responds to that symbol. Become aware of how closely the symbol fits or matches the felt sense. Go back and forth between the two of them until there is a satisfying sense of rightness – or at least as close as is possible at that time.

- As you do this you may notice that your bodily felt sense may shift and release a little. This may lead you to a deeper level, to find an even deeper match between the felt sense and the symbol.

Step 5. Sensing more deeply

You may now want to sense the felt sense more deeply. For example, you may want to find out:

- What does it need?

- How does it need me to be with it?

- What is the worst of this?

- How does it feel from its point of view?

Anything that arises should come from the felt sense rather than from your mind. Again, this may take some time. If a question is answered quickly it may not be arising from the felt sense. You could wait for a deeper sense of an answer.

Step 6. Receiving and finding a place to stop

- Whatever changes have come to you, just receive them. Depending on what they are you may want to go through the steps above a number of times before you feel that the session is completed.

- When you wish to finish the session it is best to do so gently. There will be some moments in this process when there is more activity and other times when there is less. Allow your body to tell you when it is at a resting place and it is a good time to stop.

- If you want to explore more later on, you may wish to let the bodily felt sense know that you are willing to come back if it wants you to.

- You may want to say an internal thank you for all that has come to you in the session.

In time these steps may overlap, but initially, for best results, keep them clearly separated. You may not complete all the steps in one session but may still experience an internal change. Some people prefer to practise Focusing alone, while others find it easier to do this with a companion who can facilitate the process.[15]

> **Action Box**
>
> The six steps of Focusing are:
>
> - Finding what wants your attention.
> - Getting a bodily 'felt sense' of the whole problem.
> - Symbolizing.
> - Resonating.
> - Sensing more deeply.
> - Receiving and finding a place to stop.
>
> You may like to find out about Focusing from the internet or a book, or go on a Focusing course to learn more.

Dealing with writer's block

A friend recently used Focusing when he was unable to write an academic paper. As the hand-in time drew closer he grew increasingly stressed. He couldn't get down to writing and found himself doing anything (including his tax returns!) to avoid it. When he focused on the problem, he had a 'felt sense' of something murky and unclear in his stomach area. It felt 'almost as if there is nothing but a blank space in there'. He sat with it and described it some more, haltingly at first. The words 'unclear' and then 'insubstantial' arose but he knew these weren't quite right. The feeling inside did start to change, however, and became clearer. He said, 'It's now more like a brown muddy pool.' Next the words 'a mess' came up. This still wasn't quite right but these descriptive words told him that he was on the right track.

In time, having stayed with the bodily sense, he suddenly got the word 'insufficient'. He felt a shift in his body indicating that this was important. He felt a resonance between the felt sense and the word 'insufficient'. It was a match. He asked, 'What makes this so insufficient?' and he waited. From the felt sense the answer arose. He didn't feel up to writing the paper as he thought others were more knowledgeable and could do it better. He felt a sigh of relief and his body relaxed. He knew that this was what had been stopping him from writing. Instead of feeling hopeless, he felt buoyant.

This is very common when people use Focusing successfully. They may discover something that seems very negative but they have a sense of relief. They feel better that it is now in their consciousness rather than hidden inside. Funnily enough he now felt able to write. The next day my friend sat down and started to write the paper with ease, finishing it with no further hiccups.

41 Learn from your difficulties

Interestingly, the Chinese word for 'crisis' is made up of two characters, one meaning 'danger', the other meaning 'opportunity'. Embedded within the Chinese language and culture is the belief that opportunity arises out of our difficulties. By believing this, we can start to feel positive about our ability to deal with any situation.

A simple procedure that can be used to develop this viewpoint is learning to 'reframe' whatever situations come our way. This will in turn develop our good feelings about ourselves. Mistakes literally become opportunities to learn and difficulties seen as opportunities for change. We might then find out that there is 'no failure, only feedback'.[16] We feel better about ourselves as we begin to learn from our mistakes. Try repeating this simple sentence to yourself every time you are in difficulty:

• What can I learn from this?

So, 'an error of judgement' can turn into an opportunity for greater under-standing. If we do something 'wrong', the wrongdoing can become something we can change next time around. The more we ask ourselves, 'What can I learn from this?' the more we see ourselves in a positive light. Instead of feeling you are a person who does things badly, makes mistakes and is generally 'not good enough' you can become a person who feels good about who you are, and you learn from your circumstances.

Learning from past events helps us to resolve any emotional blocks resulting from them. If we do not learn from them, similar situations will bring up the same feelings again and again. An emotional 'pattern' occurs. We may often blame other people who have said or done things that bring up these emotions, but the more we take responsibility for our lives, the more we realize that we are reacting because we have unhealed emotional wounds.

Action Box

Repeat this simple sentence to yourself whenever you are in difficulty:

* What can I learn from this?

Remember that every difficulty can become an opportunity for greater understanding.

42 Use talking therapy

Linda Chih-Ling Koo, in her book *Nourishment of Life* about life in Chinese society, wrote that:

> The traditional family structure served to provide support for the individual. Personal secrets were frequently solely shared between siblings or cousins . . . between husbands and wives and between grandparents and children. These conversational and intimate exchanges allowed family members to release emotional tensions, to have disputes settled by a third party family member and to reaffirm their self worth because of the emphatic feelings expressed by their confidante.[17]

When we are angry, sad, fearful or grief-stricken there is nothing better than being able to talk to another person in order to release our deeply held feelings. Afterwards, we often feel much better just for having talked.

The most important part of 'talking therapy' is to find a listener who will hear us without giving advice. Once our problem is out in the open and we feel heard, we may understand it better and it may recede on its own.

One patient told me that she finds it incredibly relieving and reassuring to know that someone else knows about her difficulties. It reduces the scale of the problem and puts it in perspective. Once she's told someone about it and knows she's been heard, the problem instantly feels more manageable and she can cope with it. Another patient said that when she's feeling tired and the tiredness doesn't get better after a rest, she knows there's an unexpressed emotion that needs to be teased out. She often does this by talking it through with friends. Generally the problem then blows through easily.

People in China often won't talk to 'strangers' about their problems. In the West, where family ties are less strong, we may visit a counsellor or therapist. Alternatively, it may be enough to talk to a friend.

Action Box

Bear these points in mind when choosing someone to talk to:

- Make sure that you trust the person. If you suspect that they may give away your deepest secrets then you will be unable to open up to them.
- Only talk to someone you have rapport with and who can understand you.
- The person must be able to listen to you without giving you a 'solution'.
- You may like advice sometimes. Make an agreement with the listener that they will only give advice or a solution if you specifically ask for it.

43 Use writing therapy

Sometimes it's hard to talk about our problems, so why not write them out? Writing can help us to resolve feelings or thoughts that have become stuck in our consciousness – especially if we find it difficult to talk about them.

> **Action Box**
>
> Here is one useful way of writing about our feelings:
>
> * Find a place to write where you'll be comfortable and won't be disturbed.
> * Write about your situation or problem for about 10–15 minutes continuously – don't think about your writing style or grammar.
> * Completely let go and say anything and everything you want.
> * Explore the whole situation. Write about it objectively (what actually happened) as well as subjectively (your feelings from your point of view).
> * Feel free to let out your deepest feelings. Don't plan to show anyone else – it will affect your ability to say whatever you want – make *yourself* your audience.

After writing, you may feel relieved and immediately better or you may feel a little depressed or sad for a while. Don't worry about any negative feelings – they'll pass within an hour or two and are likely to be replaced by a new perspective on your life.

You can keep what you have written in the form of a journal or diary. Alternatively you can throw the letter or writing away or even make a ritual of burning the paper to show you have cleansed the problem from your psyche.

44 The importance of positive goals

Buddhist monks who meditated in the Tien Tai mountains in the Shixuan province of China hundreds of years ago had a specific method of dealing with their negative emotions during meditation. If negative thoughts came into their heads while they were meditating they would become conscious of these thoughts – then think of something that was opposite.

For example, if they were thinking negatively about someone, they would find something about them that was positive, or if they were thinking about something that was a problem for them they would try to imagine it solved in the future. By doing this they could once more find tranquillity in their meditation.[18]

Like the Tien Tai monks, we too can find ways to retrain our mind to think positively. One way of doing this is by constructing positive goals for ourselves.

If we listen to the recurring thoughts that go through our heads we will find some that come back persistently. These could be thoughts such as 'I'll never get what I want in life', 'Don't trust anybody – they'll only let you down' or 'I always fail at everything I do'. Negative thoughts tend to become self-fulfilling prophecies, bringing with them emotional turmoil and possible ill-health.

Sometimes just one negative thought can be at the root of many negative experiences but we may be unaware of the thought. For example you may think 'The good times will all go wrong', and as a result you notice that every time you are enjoying yourself or doing something successfully you feel anxious and unsettled but don't know why. You may often be aware of your negative thoughts but find it difficult to stop them. If you are aware that you have a recurring negative thought, it can be useful to try to turn it into a positive outcome or goal.

Six steps to constructing a positive goal

Our world is a manifestation of our thoughts. If we think negatively we will have negative experiences in our lives; if we think positively our life will become more positive. Recognizing our negative thoughts is the first step to translating them into something more positive.

Sometimes we already have an idea of what we want, but wish to fine-tune it. Setting the goal and repeating it to ourselves will enable us to imagine what it will be like when we have what we want.

These are the golden rules to help us to construct a positive goal:

1. **Keep it in the present**. Rather than saying, 'I will be successful', it is better to say, 'I *am* successful'. If this sounds too strong we might soften the sentence by saying, 'I *allow myself* to be successful'. If the goal is not stated in the present it will continue to be in the future so will probably never happen.

2. **Keep it positive**. Do not construct a sentence that contains a negative word such as 'not' or 'no'. This is because the mind does not translate a negative word. The mind always thinks in pictures. For example, if we say, 'I don't have insomnia', we can't picture it. On the other hand if we say, 'I allow myself to have deep and nourishing sleep at night', we can picture ourselves deeply asleep at the end of the day.

3. **Keep it simple and achievable**. A goal that has too many parts becomes complicated and is less likely to manifest. For example, if we say, 'I allow myself to have a good job, a house, a car and a good relationship', we are diluting the possibilities of achieving any of these things. If we stop to think about what's behind wanting these things and realize, for example, that we expect them to bring us contentment and peace, then it might be better to say 'I have the things which bring me contentment and peace'. It is then more likely that we will get what we want rather than what we *think* we want.

4. **Put yourself in the goal**. If you have a picture or sense of yourself achieving the goal it is best that this shows you having achieved it, in order for it to manifest. For example, if you want to buy a new pair of trousers it is best to see yourself wearing the trousers. If you see the trousers but you are not wearing them they might be in a shop waiting for you but you might never find them!

5. **Focus on the end result not on the process of doing it**. Staying with the example above, if you imagine yourself shopping for trousers, you might wander around the shops all day but never find the pair of trousers you want. On the other hand if you see yourself wearing the new trousers you are more likely to get the outcome you desire.

Once you have constructed your outcome:

6. **Consider what might happen if you did get the goal you desire**. Think about both the negative and the positive implications. If, for example, you state, 'I allow myself to meet the person of my dreams', this might have many unwanted repercussions. The person of your dreams might live in another country, continually be unfaithful or have some bad habits you didn't predict. Think carefully about your goal and choose the wording with care!

Once you have completed the six steps above, you will have constructed a positive outcome for yourself. You might remember it by repeating it to yourself or writing it down. As you go over your goal it is useful to imagine what it will be like when you have it, as vividly as possible.

Action Box

These are the golden rules to help us to construct a positive goal.

- Keep it in the present.
- Keep it positive.
- Keep it simple and achievable.
- Put yourself in the goal.
- Focus on the end result not on the process of doing it.
- Once you have constructed your outcome consider what might happen if you achieved the goal you desire.

To fine-tune your goal even more, you can take it one step further.

Release your negative thoughts

Sometimes we construct a positive goal but find that our mind is still holding on to an underlying negative belief.

For example, you may have constructed a goal, 'I allow myself to have the perfect job for me'. You then imagine what it will be like to be working in the perfect job and make it as real as possible. Check to see if any thoughts are coming up that are contrary to this, for example, 'I won't be able to – there are no jobs in this town'. You can welcome this thought and say to yourself, 'I acknowledge that I think I won't be able to find the perfect job as there are no jobs in town, but I'm choosing to let this thought go'. Then consciously release it from your mind. Picture once more how it will be when you have this goal, and repeat the process until you feel confident that you can have this goal manifest in your life.

Action Box

The following is a way of releasing negative thoughts you are holding on to:

*   Think of your positive goal and imagine what it's like to have it.
*   Check for any thought that comes up that is contrary to you having what you want.
*   Welcome the thought.
*   Acknowledge that you have the right to have your goal and release the negative thought.

Repeat the procedure until the negative thoughts are cleared.

45 Release your blocked feelings

Expressing your emotions

Blocked emotions often occur if it is difficult or inappropriate to express them when they arise. We can remain feeling tense and frustrated or on the brink of tears. Stuck emotions cause the *qi* to stop moving inside us. Physical activity allows the energy to move again, and as a result the emotional feelings then become less intense. All emotions need to be acknowledged, including joy and good feelings, but the emotions most often held back are anger, grief and sadness.

In part of Taiwan an interesting method of expressing emotions was developed. Individuals would go to a secluded spot in the early hours of the morning and laugh, scream, shout, cry or talk to no one in particular. This would allow them to release their pent-up feelings so that the stuck *qi* could begin to circulate again. After several minutes they felt more relaxed and calm and equilibrium was restored to their systems.[19]

If emotions are stuck inside us we can try this method to release them, if we can find a place where we can cry, shout, scream and generally release our emotions. We may not realize that we are bottling up our feelings, but we do know that we are not moving forward in life. For some it can be difficult to let the feelings out. In this case, physical activity can also help us to clear stuck emotions.

Move your emotions with activity

Activity can be anything: going for a run or a vigorous walk, playing tennis or other racquet games, skipping or even jumping up and down or stamping the feet. Banging on drums can also be a useful way of releasing feelings, or beating a cushion with the fists. I have heard that some workplaces in Japan even have a punch-bag outside the washroom. The workers can hit it to release any frustration – then continue with their work in a more positive frame of mind!

To induce unshed tears we can watch a weepy film or read a moving book. As we start to cry we can free up the stuck tears and sadness.

Dealing with the root cause

Clearing emotions can be an important release, but they will recur unless we also deal with the underlying causes. We can be angry for many reasons: not feeling appreciated, feeling frightened, not feeling respected or feeling unloved. Forgiveness can be an essential ingredient for resolving anger – otherwise it may never be fully cleared.

> **Action Box**
>
> Activity can sometimes be a useful way to release blocked emotions.
>
> * Go for a run or a vigorous walk.
> * Play tennis or other racquet games.
> * Skip, jump up and down or stamp the feet.
> * Bang on drums or beat a cushion
> * Use a punch-bag!
>
> Remember that clearing emotions can be an important release, but they will recur unless we also deal with the underlying causes.

46 Get help when you need it

You may feel too unwell to deal with your emotional condition on your own. In this case you may choose to seek the support of a counsellor or therapist or find other professional help. An alternative choice may be to go to visit an acupuncturist, herbalist or another practitioner of Chinese medicine.

One patient, aged 39 with three children, found that acupuncture changed every area of her life. Before she had acupuncture she didn't feel close to her children and always used to push them away. Since having treatment she feels new love and closeness to them. Her marriage is also stronger. Before having treatment she described how she often got 'uppity' with her husband and that this was worse when she was premenstrual. Now one week before her period she only feels a little stressed. She says that having treatment changed her outlook completely.

Although she now feels different, she also knows that she needs to look after her lifestyle to remain healthy. She described to me how she used to grab anything for her meals. Now she stops and gives herself a break rather than eating on the run. She also takes much more warm food instead of just grabbing a sandwich, and drinks more water and less coffee. She says she notices that things taste better and there's an amazing difference in her skin and hair. She also walks as much as she can. She says: 'It's given me so much confidence I can walk into a room and not give a damn.'

When we are ill, our emotions easily become out of balance. We know that when a baby is sick it cries and becomes fretful or irritable. In the same way we become easily upset or irritated when we are unwell. Chinese medicine treatment positively affects our *qi*, allowing us to become healthier physically, mentally and spiritually.

The healthier we become, the better we can deal with any new difficulties. If we are unhealthy, we are often at the mercy of the emotions we feel. When we are healthy, we feel strong enough to find new ways of dealing with life events instead of reacting from our negative patterns.

Action Box

Sometimes we need the additional help of a practitioner. If you aren't coping well with your emotions an alternative choice may be to visit an acupuncturist, herbalist or another practitioner of Chinese medicine.

5 Secrets of Balancing Work, Rest and Exercise

The balance of work, rest and exercise

When I was in China I was fascinated by the way people work, rest and exercise. In the early morning large numbers of people go to the parks to practise *tai ji quan* or *qigong*[1] exercises. These exercises are designed to exercise the mind as well as the body. Those not out in the parks may be exercising inside their homes. Most people have their own favourite healthy routine and their practice prepares them for the day ahead.[2]

Having exercised, many Chinese cycle to work. In urban areas, thousands of Chinese people join the bicycle 'rush hour' in the morning. Cycling gives them vigorous exercise and is a healthy way of getting to work.

Later, in the middle of the day, it's common for them to take a short nap after they've eaten their lunch. Like people in Mediterranean countries, the Chinese people know the benefits of a long break for lunch. Workers fall asleep in their carts, office workers put their heads down at their desks and the elderly doze on roadside seats. After lunch and a rest they are ready and fresh for work in the afternoon.

As well as this lunch-break siesta, rest time is also taken after work. About two-thirds of the day is spent working and one-third relaxing. This relaxation time is spent socializing with friends, playing with the children, having a gentle walk, reading or taking the midday nap described above. Some of this rest time is spent unwinding before going to bed.

Chinese people tend to go to bed fairly early. The hours before midnight give them their most nourishing sleep. At least eight hours of deep sleep is strengthening to the organs and replenishes the reserves of energy. They then rise early in the morning ready to exercise.

Chinese medicine tells us that we need to alternate our work, relaxation and exercise and to get enough sleep. Finding a routine that balances these aspects of our life will enable us to become healthier and more contented with our lives.

In this chapter we will consider our work, relaxation, sleeping habits and how we exercise.

47 Balance *yin* and *yang* in your work and rest

The Chinese concept of balance comes from the famous *yin–yang* symbol shown in Figure 6. *Yin* and *yang* describe two energies in our lives that are constantly interacting. *Yang* is active, warm and moving in nature, while *yin* is passive, cool and calm. Although these two energies are opposites they also depend on each other.

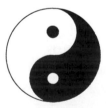

Figure 6. The *yin–yang* symbol.

Many Westerners have lifestyles that are out of balance. Some are mentally over-stressed or physically overactive – their lifestyle is too *yang*. Others have a lifestyle that is underactive and static, or *yin*. When activity and rest in our life are out of harmony we may become discontented, tired and unhealthy.

Ideally we need to balance our work, relaxation, exercise and sleep within each 24-hour cycle. This means not working for weeks at a time without a break, nor over-exercising until we are exhausted.

Some people have a lifestyle that is either too *yin or* too *yang*, while others have a mixture of underactivity and overactivity together. You may drive to work when you could walk, in order to have more time to work harder. Or you may spend time feeling exhausted and inactive then over-ride this with frenetic activity and staying up too late in order to catch up. Any extreme is unhealthy and is better avoided and replaced by a more balanced routine. Let's take a closer look at overactivity and underactivity.

A *yang* lifestyle

As success becomes ever more important, health can become less important. Many people overwork in ways they never did before. As well as paying for the mortgage and other expenses, 'work' for some people is a source of status and self-esteem. Others fear losing their job or missing a well-deserved promotion if they are off sick. We are not making time to look after our health.

Staying late at work and eating meals on the run have become part of the work ethic. We may also be combining this with juggling childcare. Work can become a sort of addiction and we may feel guilty about stopping and resting.

Action Box

Is your life too *yang* and overactive? Do you:

- Work through your lunch-break without stopping?
- Override feelings of tiredness and carry on working?
- Feel obliged to work late?
- Go back to work before you have fully recovered from illness?
- Continually juggle so many things that you never stop?

If you answered 'yes' to three or more of these questions then stop . . . you are probably in the habit of overworking, and it may be difficult for you to slow down and take notice of your health.

Suggestions
Make time to look at your daily routine. Check that you're getting enough rest, breaks at work and time to nourish yourself. Book at least a small amount of rest time into your day.

A *yin* lifestyle

While overwork is on the increase, exercise is on the decrease. Startling research shows that even children are increasingly less active than they once were. Research carried out in Bristol tracked the health of more than 14,000 children in south-west England.[3]

It found that fewer than 1 in 200 of 11-year-old girls get enough exercise. Boys were slightly more active, but still only 5% achieved the recommended daily level of physical activity.

To be healthy and stave off the risk of obesity and related conditions such as diabetes, youngsters are recommended to take an hour a day of moderate to vigorous exercise. Overall, only 2.5% of children do so. It is a sobering thought that children's activity levels peak at around the age of 11 and decline sharply during adolescence.

For adults, physical work has now largely been replaced by desk jobs. Perhaps you sit at a computer every day, drive to work and when you get home feel too tired to do anything and just sit and watch television. This inactivity can easily lead to weight gain and the vicious cycle of increased sluggishness. We need to create time to exercise. (For more about this, see the secrets later in this chapter.)

Action Box

Is your life too *yin* and static? Do you:

- Spend a large proportion of the day sitting?
- Feel tired even though you've been inactive?
- Drive to work when you could cycle or walk?
- Exercise less than once a week?
- Often feeling sluggish and a bit depressed?

If you answer is 'yes' to three or more of these questions, then you need to assess ways of bringing exercise and activity into your day.

Suggestions

You may not be able to take exercise while you are working, but try to put time aside out of working hours to take some activity.

Note: If you have had a virus from which you have never recovered or if your energy is extremely depleted then the above advice does not apply because you may have a post-viral condition. In this case visit a practitioner of Chinese medicine for specific advice. Also read Secret 48.

48 Convalescence – the forgotten secret

Convalescence is the time of recovery when the body regains its strength and health. This period begins when symptoms of the illness have disappeared, yet the body still feels weak and tired. It ends when the body's energy has been restored. It used to be a normal stage of recovery.

By taking time to recuperate we prevent other more serious conditions from occurring. We ignore our body messages at our peril. Chronic fatigue or post-viral syndrome is on the increase in Western society and this will continue until we go back to the convalescing habits of our predecessors.

Becoming ill always carries a message with it. If we are overworking that message can be that our body wants us to stop. It is increasingly common for people to feel guilty if they take time off work through sickness, and they may go back to work before they have fully regained their health.

One patient, aged 30, overworked, became ill and didn't convalesce. A benign lump was found on her spine but she went back to work before she'd even been signed off. 'I thought I was indispensable! I think I depleted my energy even more in a negative way. My body did compensate and I could keep going but I was "running on empty".' Later she became ill with breast cancer. 'This time I took March to October off work.' During this time off she reassessed her lifestyle and decided to change her stressful job.

Another common pattern is that people continue to work hard with the remains of an infection or virus in their system, with the result that the body can become so weak that it can't throw the infection off. In an extreme situation the whole system can give up and the body is unable to work at all. This can be the beginning of a post-viral condition.

A patient aged 45 is typical of this. She had periods of overworking for eight years in a demanding and stressful job in education. When she became ill with glandular fever she did not realize the importance of rest and kept working. 'If I was away no one else would do it.' She was also encouraged to exercise while still ill. Now she realizes that she should have been resting. 'The final straw was having a hysterectomy and not resting for long enough afterwards. I never recovered and got ME.'[4]

When we are ill we easily become tired because our body tells us it needs to rest in order to recover. Many of us have lost touch with these messages and no longer realize the importance of convalescing. Had this patient known to rest when she was initially ill she thinks she would be healthy today.

Action Box

Consider these aspects of convalescence

- Next time you have an infection don't go into work and spread it to others. Rest for the time you're infectious then take one more day off to recuperate and regain your strength.
- If you are severely ill take plenty of time off so that your body can regain its strength and health. You might choose to use the time that you take to convalesce to examine why you have become ill and make any changes necessary to prevent further illness.
- As well as resting, make sure you eat healthily during the time of convalescence.
- Don't exercise while you're ill – especially if you have an infection.
- While convalescing you may find that even mild activity tires you mentally and physically. A small amount of exercise can sometimes be helpful but be aware of how your body responds. Take note of how much you can exercise and how much you need to stop and rest.
- Remember that susceptibility to further illness and infection is very high after you have been ill. Exposure to the elements can result in further infection, which prolongs recuperation time (see Chapter 6).

49 After a miscarriage, take time to rest

Chinese medicine teaches that after a miscarriage (or abortion) is also a time to convalesce We know that pregnancy can be depleting for a women, but a miscarriage or abortion can be more so. This is because the natural cycle of pregnancy has been cut short. A woman often goes through huge psychological and physical adjustments following a miscarriage. Her instinct may be to become pregnant again as soon as possible to make up for the loss. A healthier option for her is to rest and recover from the grief.

After an abortion a woman may assume that she can go back to normality immediately. Months later, at the time when the baby would have been born, depression can set in. In this case the would-be mother often doesn't make the connection or realize that her body and mind are grieving and adjusting to the loss of the child.

This happened to one of my patients. She came for treatment saying she was very depressed and didn't understand why. She wasn't consciously thinking too much about the abortion she had had nine months before but her body hadn't forgotten. Now it was time for the birth, and depression had set in. After acupuncture treatment and rest, she started to adjust and gradually felt much healthier and able to cope again.

If a woman becomes pregnant again before she is ready, she may become more depleted and tired, or the baby may be less healthy. Allow at least six months or even a year to recover from a miscarriage. This should enable a woman to fully regain her energy and overcome the loss fully.

Action Box

This is for those who have lost a baby. If you have had a miscarriage, have you properly recovered? Did you rest and allow yourself to grieve afterwards? Some people have a ritual for the lost baby, which helps them to say a proper goodbye. Many feel this enables its spirit to move on and the parent(s) to move on as well. The ceremony may be quite simple, like reading out a meaningful poem, singing a specially chosen song or spending time in meditative silence or prayer. The main purpose is that it's special and meaningful to you.

---

50 The positive effects of fulfilling work

Is your work enjoyable and worthwhile? If we have a job that we enjoy doing and find fulfilling then this has positive effects on our health. A small amount of stress can be stimulating but extreme stress will drain our internal resources. Unfulfilling or very boring work may also have negative consequences on our health.

Even if you don't like your job, try to bring as many nourishing activities as possible into your day to lift yourself. Use ideas from this chapter or from Chapter 4 on emotions. The healthier we are and the better we feel in ourselves, the more we can enjoy what we do and feel less stressed by it. Looking after your lifestyle may enable you to find more fulfilment from your job. Sometimes changing your job may turn out to be the best decision. Feeling healthier should enable you to make the right choice.

One way of dealing with stress and generating good feelings is called practising your inner smile.

Action Box

Practise your inner smile

This well-known Chinese exercise takes only a few minutes to do. It relaxes and rejuvenates the internal organs and helps us through any tense situation. This exercise can be done at any time – in the office, in a stressful meeting or when studying for exams. It will make any difficulties easier to cope with.

- Sit with your back straight.
- Imagine something that will make you smile. It could be a beautiful picture, relaxing music or a good feeling generated by some enjoyable event. As you think of it allow yourself to smile internally – it doesn't have to be visible – only felt by you.
- Allow the smile to shine out of your eyes.
- Now let the smile travel downwards into your internal organs. Notice the feeling of relaxation generated by the internal smile.
- Allow the smile to travel all the way down to your belly and feel the stability it gives you.
- Carry on with what you are doing, keeping the feeling generated by the internal smile.

Others will also respond to the good feelings activated by this internal smile.

51 Keep your life regular

We are generally creatures of habit and it is better to have a habitual lifestyle than to live a chaotic one. A study carried out on 7,000 people from the 1960s to the 1990s at the University of California School of Public Health backs this up.[5]

It found that many unhealthy lifestyle practices affected a person's wellbeing. Some of these practices, such as tobacco and alcohol intake, were obvious, as were others such as physical inactivity. The biggest surprise, however, was the effect of an irregular lifestyle. Someone who was teetotal and didn't smoke was still more likely to die prematurely or to suffer from disabling illnesses if they had irregular habits such as eating between meals, having irregular sleep or skipping breakfast. The researchers came to the conclusion that a regular lifestyle is one of the main ways we can maintain our health.

Besides not smoking or drinking alcohol, some of the regular good habits that were found to affect a person's wellbeing were:

- eating regular meals

- having a good breakfast

- getting regular moderate exercise

- getting enough sleep

- eating so as to maintain a moderate weight.

Chinese medicine stresses the importance of balance in everything we do. While not wanting to become rigid, keeping our lives regular could make a lasting difference.

Action Box

A practical step to help you to lead a regular life is to make modifications that are so simple that they easily become habitual. If you find you are getting benefit from them you will naturally integrate them into your life and do them regularly. For example, go to bed at a regular time or set a time to have your lunch or evening meal. Stick to this time, but without becoming rigid as there will be some exceptions in certain circumstances.

52 Points to relieve smoker's cravings

We all know that smoking is associated with many illnesses including lung cancer, asthma, bronchitis, heart disease and emphysema. Research shows that being a non-smoker has a significant effect on our longevity and wellbeing (see Secret 51 and research on page 117).

Much help exists to support you if you want to give up smoking, including books, hypnotism and nicotine patches. Acupuncture, using points on the ear, can be extremely beneficial. Whatever way you choose, you must be ready to stop smoking. Ask yourself the questions in the Action Box to help yourself prepare.

You can massage to relieve cravings while you are giving up. Lightly press or massage one of the four points in Figure 4 if you feel a craving, whichever one helps to relieve the craving most.

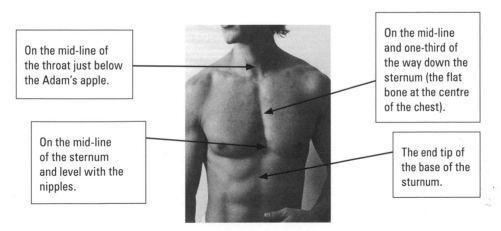

On the mid-line of the throat just below the Adam's apple.

On the mid-line and one-third of the way down the sternum (the flat bone at the centre of the chest).

On the mid-line of the sternum and level with the nipples.

The end tip of the base of the sturnum.

Figure 4. Massage points for relieving cravings.

Action Box

Questions to ask yourself before giving up smoking

These questions may be useful if you are thinking about giving up smoking. They can also apply to any other addiction:

- Do I really want to give up smoking? No treatment will work unless you are really motivated to give it up.
- In what circumstances do I smoke? During tea breaks, while driving, after eating, when you are upset or a combination of many other situations.
- What do I get from smoking? For example, 'it warms my chest', 'it relaxes me', 'it's just a habit', 'it gives me a break' or 'it stops me feeling frustrated'. Your answer may be one or a combination of these.
- Knowing what smoking does for me, what can I do to replace it? For example, activities such as 'relaxing with a book', 'breathing exercises', 'chewing gum', 'going for a walk' or 'giving myself a treat such as . . .'
- What benefits will I gain from giving it up? For example, 'I won't cough any more', 'I'll smell better', 'I'll save money' or 'I'll prove that I have will power'.
- When will I be ready to stop? Decide on a 'D' day. Having a realistic date in the future helps you to plan ahead for how you will give up. Alternatively you may be ready to stop immediately.

53 Exercise while you work

In the past people used to exercise while doing their daily work or travelling to or from work more than they do today. Our habits have changed dramatically.

Labouring and farming jobs once involved a lot of physical work which has now been replaced by machinery. Daily housework was also a fairly active occupation. No one would want to go back to the days before labour-saving devices such as vacuum cleaners and washing machines, but if we did, we would certainly be more active. Cycling or walking to work was also the norm at one time, while today we drive even short distances.

Bring exercise into your life

There are many different ways to bring physical exercise into your life. Gill, 49, takes her dog for a walk in Richmond Park for 40 minutes a day. 'Walking doesn't sound exciting but my tension levels abate. There's a certain briskness in my step and I walk up a hill for extra exercise.' Judy, 37, goes horse-riding. 'It's the one thing I absolutely always do twice a week regardless of how busy I am.' She's done it for the past six years and finds it really good for relaxing her and switching off her mind. Margi, who is in her 40s, says she both cycles and walks. She doesn't have a car and is fitter now than she has been for years. 'For a period of my life I was really tired. Before I'd look at a hill and think, oh no! I would never exercise as I thought it was too much effort. But once I started I could do it easily.'

Action box

Try these ways to bring exercise into your daily life:

- Jog to the shops.
- Walk upstairs rather than taking a lift.
- Park some distance from the office and walk.
- Cycle to work.
- Go out dancing.
- Gardening.

An exercise DVD may also help you to structure a routine. Choose carefully, and whatever you choose, make it enjoyable!

Studies have found that regular exercise helps to improve your energy and significantly lower levels of anger, depression and tension.[6] Regular exercise throughout your life can also help to prevent osteoporosis.[7]

In addition, exercise has been proved to decrease the risk of heart disease. In 1980 a questionnaire evaluated the daily physical activity of 17,944 middle-aged British civil servants. Eight years later a follow-up survey was taken. It was found that the incidence of heart disease was 50% less in those who had a more active lifestyle.[8]

54 Walk your way to health

A famous Chinese text, the *Lao, Lao Heng Yan*, has a special section on walking. It points out that walking relaxes the muscles and tendons, strengthens the limbs, promotes digestion and calms the mind.[9] Modern research backs this up. A study at Loughborough University found that walking at a low, even intensity caused people to burn fat and lose weight.[10]

Another study, conducted by the Department of Medicine, Harvard Medical School and Brigham and Women's Hospital, Boston, MA, compared walking with vigorous exercise in relation to the incidence of coronary heart disease. The study was carried out on 72,488 female nurses who were aged between 40 and 65 in 1986.

The results showed that women who walked for three hours per week at a brisk pace were 30–40% less likely to be at risk from heart problems than those who didn't exercise. Walking was just as beneficial to the women's health as other more vigorous exercise. Women who become active later in life also have a lower risk of heart problems than those who remain sedentary.[11]

Other studies have found that the effects gained from walking can be accumulated throughout the day and just 30 minutes a day can reduce blood fats and increase the body's ability to burn fat.[12] In fact three 10-minute walks can be as effective as one continuous 30-minute session and can also reduce stress, tension and anxiety.[13]

Studies show that walking slows the ageing process, prevents coronary heart disease, cuts the risk of strokes, reduces cancer risks and improves cancer survival rates, helps to control blood glucose in type 2 diabetes, boosts your mood and lifts depression.[14]

From a Chinese medicine perspective, walking stimulates the movement of *qi* in our body and gives us energy. There are two 'gates' in the feet that are affected when we walk. The first is in the heel and lies towards the centre and rear of the heel. The second is in the ball of the foot where there is an acupuncture point (see page 125) that is stimulated.[15]

As we walk on the heel *qi* naturally falls down and through our body into the earth. This helps to clear blocked or stagnant *qi*. Putting pressure on the ball of the foot allows *qi* to flow from the earth up into our legs and body. This gives us *qi* to use in our daily life.[16]

Action Box

Ten useful tips to help you to walk to health[17]

- Don't take a big stride when you walk – walk at a natural pace.
- Wear comfortable shoes that fit correctly – there is no point in walking in shoes that are too tight or don't support your feet.
- Walk from heel to toe in flowing movements – the two energy gates described above will be activated when you walk this way.
- Swing your arms as you walk – bend your arms and let them swing to counter balance your leg motion.
- Don't let your arms cross the centre line or come up further than your chest.
- Look ahead as you walk. Your eyes should focus about 20–30 yards ahead.
- Do not lean too far back or forward – walk upright.
- Wear the right clothing – it should be light, layered and made from natural fibres that can breathe.
- Don't allow yourself to become dehydrated. Drink at least one cup of water every 20 minutes.
- Enjoy your walking! Give yourself a rest when you need it and take note of the 70% rule! (see page 136).

---

55 Sleep – the best natural cure

Having a regular seven to eight hours of sleep each night is important for our overall health. Nowadays feeling tired all the time is quite common. If you are constantly exhausted, are you getting enough sleep? Sleep eliminates fatigue and restores health. An old Chinese saying claims that 'to sleep well is better than to eat well'.[18] It rightly asserts that even nourishing food and tonics cannot replace the role of sleep.

An intriguing study of 8,000 people aged 35 to 55, who were followed over a number of years, found that those who slept for seven to eight hours a night had the lowest risk of cardiovascular-related problems. The less sleep the greater the risk.

Another earlier study found that less sleep was associated with all causes of death including cancer, stroke or heart disease. Remarkably it was found that short sleepers of six hours or fewer or those who consistently slept for a lot more than nine hours were 30% more likely to die prematurely.[19]

The results of these studies will not surprise those who practise Chinese medicine. During the night our *qi* withdraws inside us and nourishes our organs. If we don't get enough rest and sleep we will not replenish our *qi*. In time we will be drawing on reserves and depleting ourselves.

Although about eight hours of sleep may be normal when we are well, when we are ill it is important to rest for longer. If our *qi* has become weakened from ill-health, rest will replenish it.

We all become ill and tired at times. Sometimes the best 'cure' for our illnesses is to go to bed and sleep until we are better. I've known people who have slept for several days, with only breaks for meals, and this sleep has seemed to trigger their recovery. If we feel like sleeping for long periods this may be our body telling us that we need to rest in order to recover.

Action Box

If you have difficulty sleeping

There is nothing worse than tossing and turning and being unable to sleep. Chinese medicine suggests that before sleeping we should 'first relax the heart'. This means that we should avoid going to bed excited, nervous or overstimulated. Here are some suggestions to help you sleep better:

- Cultivate going to bed at a regular time each night – even if you don't immediately fall asleep.
- Cut out caffeine-based stimulants such as coffee and tea. Buy decaffeinated drinks or drink herbal teas and water.
- Don't engage in stimulating activities before bed. Watching television, reading exciting books or vigorous activity are all stimulating and keep us awake.
- Don't eat late at night – you will go to bed still digesting your food.
- Do a relaxation exercise (see the relaxation exercise in the Action Box on page 131), or use a relaxation tape.
- Meditate or do a gentle *qigong* exercise before bed.
- Massage your feet, especially at the acupuncture point in Figure 8. Massaging this point helps to bring excess energy from the head to the feet, thus calming the *qi* and helping us to sleep.

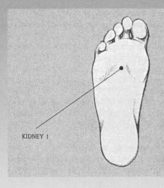

KIDNEY 1

Figure 8. Massage feet here to induce sleep.

- The Chinese medicine classic *Han Shou Yao Yan* says: 'It will be much easier to go to sleep if one washes one's feet in hot water before going to bed.'[20] This is another way to bring *qi* from the head to the feet, thus inducing a calm mind.

In addition to following the suggestions above, consider whether your diet is deficient in 'Blood'-nourishing food. If you are what the Chinese call 'Blood-deficient' you may feel unsettled inside, causing difficulty sleeping (see page 44).

For more on insomnia, see page 215. If you have chronic insomnia and these suggestions don't help, visit a Chinese medicine practitioner.

56 Sleep in a healthy posture

About one-third of your life is spent sleeping. To enable you to get the greatest health benefits from sleeping it is important that you sleep in a good posture and are relaxed. Some *qigong* practitioners suggest lying on the back so that the spine is straight and the body is unobstructed. Many long-term joint problems can develop from sleeping in awkward positions with joints tensed.

Another traditional position is to lie on your right side with the top leg bent and the other leg straight. The right hand can be placed under the head for a pillow and the left hand rests on the thigh. In this position the heart is high up and does not get constricted. The liver, which Chinese medicine says 'stores Blood', is lower down and hence receives more blood. This posture also allows our *qi* to circulate freely.

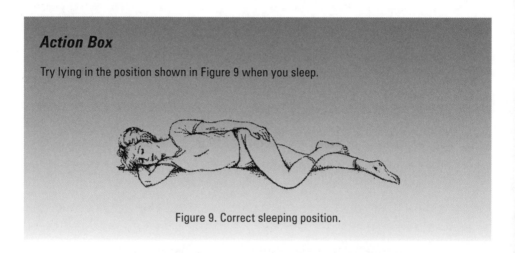

Action Box

Try lying in the position shown in Figure 9 when you sleep.

Figure 9. Correct sleeping position.

Don't use a pillow that is too high or firm, which could mean you are sleeping with your neck in a bad posture and constricting the blood flow to the head, which can cause neck problems and headaches, and even affect the eyesight.

57 Take a 'power' nap

Most Chinese people have a short rest, after their lunch, usually for no longer than half an hour. Office workers will put their heads on their desks, the elderly sleep on outside seats. Workers doze in their carts while others sleep in their cars. After the rest they are refreshed and can work with renewed vigour.

Studies confirm this to be beneficial. People who were allowed to sleep without restriction developed an interesting pattern. They began to prefer to take a nap in the middle of the day. Although they didn't always sleep, the rest left them refreshed and ready for the afternoon. Research suggests that an afternoon nap could be more in tune with our natural biological rhythms than just one long sleep at night.[21]

In another study, carried out at Harvard University, college students were challenged to detect subtle changes in an image during four different test sessions on the same day. The scores of the participants who didn't nap declined throughout the final two sessions. In contrast, volunteers who took a 30-minute nap after completing the second session showed no ensuing performance dips. What's more, those who napped for one hour responded progressively faster and more accurately in the third and fourth sessions.[22] A nap (or a good night's sleep) often leads to breakthroughs in learning or may enhance a person's capacity to learn new things.

In Japan a nap taken during the day is called *inemuri*. This literally means 'to be asleep while present'. In Japan dozing anywhere is allowed and it can even be done in business meetings – in the West, of course, this would be unacceptable.

Inemuri is viewed as exhaustion from working hard and sacrificing sleep at night – so some even fake it to look committed to their job! Strict rules apply to inemuri. These include who is allowed to do it – only those high up or low down in a company – and also how to do it – you must remain upright to show you are still socially engaged in some way.[23]

> ### Action Box
>
> Everyone has different rhythms so it is impossible to recommend how long you need for a nap. If you regularly nap you may develop a good idea about what duration works best for you as well as the best environment, equipment, position and associated factors that help to induce the best sleep. An average duration of around 20–30 minutes is often most effective in order to gain the maximum mental and physical benefits. Older people may need longer. You may take power-naps out of necessity, for example, if you regularly don't sleep well at night and are drowsy at work, and have a sleep during your lunch-break. Or you may prefer to take naps regularly even if you get a full night's sleep just because it improves your feeling of wellbeing and vitality. Try out what works best for you. Notice what effect a nap has on your daily life.

58 Make time for rest and relaxation

Relaxation is as important to our health as sleep. The pace of life in the 21st century is increasing all the time, making it difficult sometimes to make time for rest.

If you are always on the go, you might try to follow the example of one of my patients who makes sure she gets time to rest. 'In order to rest I now timetable in my relaxing time and time off.' In this way she can take time out and not worry about the fact that she's not doing things. She also looks at the balance of her working days compared with rest days and factors in time for herself – especially as she does lots of weekend work.

Action Box

There are many healthy ways of relaxing. These are some suggestions.

- Listen to a relaxation tape.
- Go out for a gentle walk in the country.
- Meditate.
- Have a massage.
- Take a relaxing bath.
- Use the flotation tank at the local spa.
- Practise *qigong* or other relaxing exercises.

Whatever you decide to do, it must be enjoyable. If it is not enjoyable, it won't be relaxing!

It is all too easy to get caught up with caring for others and never spend time nourishing ourselves. This is especially true of mothers with young children and other carers. Booking in some space for pleasurable activity, even if it is only for a short time every week, can be rejuvenating.

You may prefer to relax inside your home either by yourself or with others, or you may prefer going out for relaxation. Holidays are an important way of getting rest and relaxation. Relaxation can, of course, overlap with exercise, and those who do *qi* exercises are often pleased to find they are doing a relaxing activity that they also enjoy. Whatever you decide to do, it must be enjoyable or it won't be relaxing. Relaxation inevitably has positive repercussions on our health.

59 Scan your body to relax

Scanning the body is another way to help us to relax. It wakes up our consciousness and is an important way to gain more control over our *qi*. The deeper we go inside ourselves as we scan, the more we slow down, and the more we slow down the more we relax. Relaxation allows our *qi* to flow freely through the body so that the Organs also become invigorated and the mind more relaxed. This leads to greater health and wellbeing physically, mentally and emotionally.

Action Box

Scanning the body

Sit with your back straight or lie down with your arms and legs outstretched and your head raised on a low pillow. You may wish to place a pillow under your knees. Notice your body sensations as you relax the body down three lines:

- **Line 1:** down the two sides – the outer sides of the head – neck – shoulders – upper arms – elbows – wrists – palms – fingers.
- **Line 2:** top of the head – face – neck – chest – abdomen – thighs – knees – legs – ankles – toes.
- **Line 3:** head – back of the neck – back – waist – back of thighs – hollows of the knees – back of the legs – heels – soles of feet.

Each line will take a few minutes to complete. Having completed the three lines, focus your attention onto the lower abdomen for about one minute. Repeat the exercise as many times as you wish. [24]

At first when you practise relaxation techniques you may find that your mind easily drifts off. This is what the Chinese call a 'monkey mind' – a mind with a short attention span. Be patient with yourself, however, and you will soon start to concentrate for increasingly longer periods. This should result in better day-to-day concentration and increased peace and contentment.

Below is a relaxation exercise that can be useful for a rest in the middle of the day or as preparation for a relaxing sleep before bed. It will take you straight into the experience of relaxation.

Action Box

A simple relaxation exercise that really works!

Sit down and take off your shoes and, if you wear them, your glasses:

- Rest your palms in your lap, facing upwards.
- Gently curl your fingers and thumbs a little towards your palms and then uncurl them.
- Do these actions repeatedly in a slow, rhythmical fashion in which you never stop moving.
- Let the curl of your fingers become the uncurl and the uncurl become the curl. Usually the slower you move, the better, but 'pulse' at whatever speed feels most relaxing to you.
- Now in unison with your fingers gently curl and uncurl your toes a little. Do this in such a way that you don't tighten your toes, even if this means that you barely move them.
- Now gently close your eyes and partially open them as you curl and uncurl. Let them remain unfocused as you open and close them.
- Continue to 'pulse' your fingers, toes and eyes this way for two minutes. If you find yourself wanting to inhale and exhale with the movements, do this too.
- If other parts of your body want to let go or move a bit as well, let them.
- Play with the speed of your pulsing, but err on the side of going slower and slower. In fact, how slow can you go and still keep moving?

As you do this exercise you may find you begin to relax. This is consistent with Chinese theory, which says that rhythmical, slow, moderate and continuous movements are relaxing. Further, if you relax your hands, feet and face, then the whole of your body is likely to relax. For the next two weeks, do this little exercise each day, whenever you find that you'd like to relax. See whether and when it works for you.[25]

Exercise can be 'internal' or 'external'

Exercise is also important for our overall health and vitality. Chinese medicine distinguishes between two types of exercise – external and internal.

External exercises

External exercise is any exercise that focuses primarily on physical activity. Exercise carried out in the West is often of this type, and includes running, cycling, swimming or playing other sports. In China 'harder' style martial arts like kung fu also come into this category. External exercises emphasize strengthening the physical body and can be quite vigorous. Although they do affect our general wellbeing, there is no emphasis on the mental and spiritual aspects of a person.

Internal exercises

Internal exercises focus on movements that activate the inside of the body and the organs rather than purely external movement. These exercises tend to be gentler than external ones. *Qigong* and *tai ji quan* come under this heading, as does yoga and 'soft' martial arts like aikido. Doing these internal exercises helps us develop internal strength and become calmer and healthier from within.

Qigong

Qigong and *tai ji quan* are rapidly becoming popular in the West. *Qi* means energy and *gong* means practice. These exercises activate our *qi*. *Qigong* has a significant effect on improving health and maintaining wellbeing. It also helps us to develop mentally and spiritually and will clear stress, remove tension and promote relaxation. In general, the exercises are performed by moving in a slow and relaxed way, while at the same time maintaining a good posture, sometimes while standing still, sometimes while gently moving.

Qigong and our health

There are a number of different styles of *qigong* and every teacher will have their own unique method. If practised well, all styles will have an overall positive effect on our health and wellbeing. As far back as 200 BCE Chinese doctors realized that gentle exercise can stimulate the flow of our *qi*. When our *qi* runs smoothly throughout our bodies we remain healthy. If our *qi* is blocked or weakened this can lead to ill-health.

Some exercises improve our health in a general way by creating a better balance of *qi* throughout our system. A better balance of *qi* can also lead to greater feelings of contentment and wellbeing. Other exercises are specifically designed to improve the functioning of different organs in the body such as the Kidney, Liver, Lung or Heart. Others are aimed at other functions such as helping the digestive system, improving the circulation or clearing the head.

Research

Much research into the health benefits of *qigong* has been carried out in China and results have been very positive. In one study patients who had raised blood pressure were monitored over a period of 20 years. Half the patients practised *qigong*, and this group's blood pressure stabilized and lowered and there was a decrease in the amount of medication needed. The other half that didn't practise had an increase in blood pressure and also an increase in medication.[26]

In another study into heart function and circulation researchers evaluated the effects of *qigong* on 120 elderly patients, using ultrasonic techniques. After practising *qigong* for one year, the patients' heart output was increased and circulation improved. Only 39.1% of those practising *qigong* had circulatory problems compared with 73.9% of those not practising *qigong*.[27]

While writing this book I spoke to many people who practise *qigong*. All had different reasons for practising and had gained a variety of benefits. For example, one person said that it's part and parcel of toning her: 'It also starts up my day and gives me a focus. If I don't do it I'm all helter-skelter.' Another *qigong* colleague finds that he's looser and walks more upright. 'My chest is softer and easier and my shoulder, which has been a problem for 30 years, is enormously better. I'm over 60 and I haven't stiffened up in the way I might have.' He says it makes everything a little smoother and easier. 'I also feel more vitality from doing it and I have more comfort in my body.'

Action Box

A gentle *qigong* stretch

This exercise is a complete stretch (see Figure 10). It strengthens all the internal organs and stretches the spine to help back problems. Practising it daily will strengthen breathing and help to create a smooth flow of *qi* throughout the body:

- Stand relaxed with the feet shoulders-width apart, knees slightly bent and feet facing forwards. Place the hands about one and a half inches below the navel, palms facing downwards and with the fingers pointing towards each other.
- Breathe in knowing that you are taking pure, vital *qi* into your body. At the same time, bring the hands outwards and upwards in front of the body so that the palms are held high above the head facing upwards. Look up and at the same time stretch the palms of the hands upwards, keeping the back straight.
- Breathe out and at the same time lower the hands out to the sides while bending the knees slightly. Know that you are breathing out any stale or impure *qi* and let it clear through the fingers.
- Bring the hands back to the starting position.

Repeat this exercise at least ten times every day. You will feel the benefits if it is performed on a regular basis.

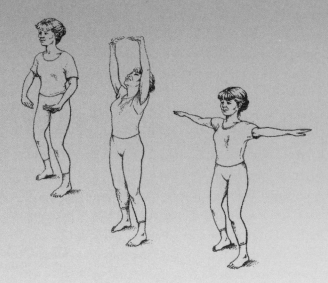

Figure 10. A *qigong* stretch.

61 Exercise according to your age, activity, build and constitution

Chinese medicine teaches that internal and external exercises are beneficial to our health and understands the need for both.

At the beginning of our lives we are normally very *yang*. *Yang* activity is very outgoing and we move from being energetic children to active adults. Later in life we naturally become more *yin* and may wish to slow down. People in the West commonly ignore this move from *yang* to *yin* energy and do not listen to their body's messages. As a result many people, especially women when they come into menopause, are overworking when they should be slowing down.

Overactivity uses up our calming and cooling *yin* energy and results in symptoms like hot flushes and feelings of agitation. A certain amount of vigorous exercise is useful earlier in life, especially if we have a strong constitution (see Chapter 2). If we are older or frailer we might prefer to do more gentle, internal exercises.

Our body type will also indicate what is the right kind of exercise for us. People with large, strong bodies can do more external exercise than those who have smaller, frailer bodies – although internal exercise is still good for them. Those with smaller body types still need activity but can do less and often prefer the internal type.

Half an hour of *qigong* practice daily is a good idea, although some people practise more. It is better to practise a small amount regularly than a larger amount at irregular times. Fifteen minutes practised every day is better than a three-hour session at irregular intervals. External exercise may be best carried out a minimum of three times a week in 20-minute sessions; activities such as walking, cycling, swimming or dancing may be preferable to more formal exercises, such as those practised at a gym.

Action Box

There is no standard amount of activity and rest. How much we need depends on our age, build and constitution and how much activity we take during the rest of the day. If our work is not balanced between mental and physical activity we can redress this imbalance by the way we exercise. For most adults, 20 to 30 minutes of external physical activity three times a week is a good minimum. Internal exercises are best practised daily. Bearing in mind your age and build, assess whether you're doing the right kind of exercise and activity.

62 Know the 70% principle for all activity

Too much exercise, internal or external, can be harmful to our health. Like overworking, exercising until you drop or being overly vigorous is more likely to deplete your energy than to improve your health.

It is best to aim to function at less than our full capacity. Chinese medicine emphasizes balance and suggests moderation in everything. Over-straining when exercising can lead to injury, tension or over-taxing your system. The net result of this is not better health – in fact you are more likely to feel worse and eventually stop the activity altogether.

My *qigong* teacher suggests that we always exercise to 70% of our capacity. He calls this 'the 70% principle'. In order to calculate the 70% principle we first need to assess our physical capacity in terms of range of movement, length of time of practice and how much we can do without actually collapsing. Once this is determined we can estimate what 70% of that activity is. The percentage is not rigid and can vary from 60 to 80%.[28] The 70% principle also applies to eating (see page 66).

It may be useful to remind yourself regularly of the 70% principle. Never push your body into activity that it doesn't wish to do or go beyond your limits. If you feel exhausted by exercise or don't enjoy doing it, then it is not right for you.

I have experienced the results of over-training in my own *qigong* practice. I once went to a teacher who encouraged his students to push themselves to their limits. I obeyed his instructions thinking this was fine for me. For some months I kept doing these exercises, then one day I stopped. Nothing enticed me to take up those exercises again. My whole body and mind had rebelled and said 'no'. In contrast I now practise to about 70% of my capacity as recommended. I have been practising this style of *qigong* for many years and continue to enjoy it.

Action Box

Carry out any exercise you normally do and notice the way you do it. Ask yourself: 'Do I go for no pain no gain, or am I more gentle on myself?' You can do any exercise with consciousness and focus and using the 70% principle.

Warning signs that your exercise routine is too strenuous may be:

- Your joints are getting very stiff and sore and don't recover.
- You find it exhausting and you remain tired for some time.
- You have to push yourself mentally to do it – your mind rebels.
- You have to push yourself physically to do it and you're testing your endurance.
- You are constantly getting injured.

---

63 Find an exercise routine

It is best to have a routine when exercising. Getting into a regular habit will mean you will continue to practise. Most people begin exercising with great enthusiasm, but maintaining the habit when the initial 'high' has gone is more of a challenge. Remember what we said earlier: it takes a month to change a habit – so stick with it. If you can exercise regularly for a month it will by then become a part of your everyday routine.

> ### Action box
>
> Points to consider when planning for a healthy routine:
>
> - Decide on how you would like to exercise and when you will do it – write this down. Make it a part of your routine.
> - Plan exercise into your day. If you have a list of things to do, put it on the list.
> - If necessary make compromises – sometimes you may need to give up an activity to make way for a healthier change. For example, you may decide to leave work earlier to go to the gym or to do *qigong* exercises before bed instead of watching television.
> - Make small changes slowly and try to incorporate them into the lifestyle you have now.
> - Do exercises that you find enjoyable. If you don't enjoy your exercises they won't benefit you – find other exercises that you like.
> - Don't over-strain or over-exercise – this leads to tension and depletes rather than enhances your *qi*.
>
> Remember that it takes a month to fully integrate changes into our lives.

64 Find a regular practice space

As part of establishing a routine, it can be useful to find a space where you can relax, exercise or do *qigong* or *tai ji* consistently. It is also helpful to create a rhythm, such as practising at the same time and for the same amount of time each day. One regular feature might be to walk to the same place and face the same direction each day. Then being in that space starts to mean practice to you, and the mere act of getting yourself to that place can help you to get 'in the mood', so to speak.

When you practise you set up energetic patterns not only in your own *qi* but also in the energy of the environment around you. If you practise in the same place every day, you'll affect the energy of that place so that it is conducive to practice. Then when you step into that place, that energy pattern will help you get started with your practice.

Ideally the place you find for your practice will feel comfortable to begin with, and be a place you inherently enjoy being in. Then going to that place will be something you naturally look forward to, and you then will associate practice with things that are enjoyable.

You don't need a whole special room in which to practise. It could be a corner or the centre of a room that you use for many other purposes. But for your practice you might always face in a direction that you don't otherwise face. Or you might put down a special rug to stand on that you only use for practice. Spend time trying out ideas like these to create a space that you dedicate to your practice.

How do you find the right place? Trust your intuition to help you find a comfortable spot. Wander among the possible spots. Face different directions. Do a little practice in each one. Try to 'feel' which spot is the most comfortable and natural for you.

Pick a spot and stick to it, even if it isn't perfect – remember the 70% principle. Then practise there regularly, even if it's just a few minutes every day.[29]

Action Box

Finding a space to practise

- Create a rhythm to practise, such as practising at the same time and for the same amount of time each day.
- Face in the same direction each day to get 'in the mood'.
- Make sure your regular spot feels comfortable to be in.
- Your 'place' might just be a corner or the centre of a room that you use for other purposes.
- You might put down a special rug that you use only for practice.
- Trust your intuition and try to feel which spot is best for you.
- Practise there regularly, even if it's just a few minutes every day.

You could also have a regular space for other activities such as writing a journal or having a 'power' nap.

65 Exercise in the 'spirit' of *qigong*

Qigong is practised by emphasizing three important principles – keeping a focused mind, maintaining good posture and staying relaxed. These are discussed below. Any exercise can be done in the 'spirit' of enhancing our *qi* if we apply these principles.

Exercising in the spirit of *qigong* is in direct contrast to the way most external exercise is carried out. Most external exercise is done with tension and speed rather than relaxation and softness. The exerciser also often pays attention only to the body rather than to the body *and* how it feels internally. Most external exercise is practised with a posture that will not enhance our *qi* flow.

Exercising in the spirit of *qigong* will enhance the quality of the exercises we do and therefore create more positive benefits from them.

All *qi* practices emphasize a focused mind, good posture and relaxation. By affecting our *qi* they balance our body, mind and spirit, which in turn leads to better health.

A focused mind

There is a saying that 'where the mind goes our *qi* follows' and this is certainly true when it comes to *qigong* practice. When we practise *qigong* the mind needs to be fully involved and at the same time relaxed and calm. With a relaxed and calm mind we can scan our bodies from top to bottom and notice areas of tension, contraction or numbness. Focusing on these areas can enable us to release any internal blockages and awaken the flow of *qi* in the body. We can also follow our breath as it goes in through the nose and down to the belly. Alternatively, an exercise may be carried out while putting the attention on the *dantien* (a place approximately three finger widths below the navel). More is written about the *dantien* in Chapter 2.

Good posture

When standing or sitting it is important that our posture is upright and the spine remains straight. Align the body so that your weight can travel downwards from the middle of the spine through the hips and into the arches of the feet. The base of the spine should point downwards towards the feet. The upper body should have a slight upward lift through the middle and upper spine and into the neck and head. The head should feel as if it is floating slightly above the neck allowing the head to be upright. The chest should be slightly hollowed but not collapsed. The better the posture the more fluidly our *qi* can flow through the system. This will in turn enhance our health and wellbeing on every level.[30] For more on standing posture see page 27, on constitution.

Relaxation

All *qi* exercises are carried out by slowing down, softening and relaxing inside. Relaxation allows the *qi* to circulate smoothly through the body. This in turn enhances our vitality. The relaxation of *qigong* and other internal exercises is very alive and dynamic because our mind is focused as we relax.

Action Box

Combining a focused mind, good posture and relaxation enhances our experience of any exercise we do. This often means we become more conscious, alert and aware and can result in improvements to our health.

Try taking just one of these principles and add it to your next session. It will enhance the quality of your exercise and you will find you finish your practice with an inner sense of wellbeing.

66 What you learn from a good teacher becomes yours for life

Basic *qi* exercises are simple and safe to do. If you wish to progress in the practice of *qigong* or *tai ji quan*, however, it is always best to do so under the guidance of an experienced teacher.

People from Eastern cultures usually have great respect for their teachers. They recognize the huge gift that is being imparted to them. Whatever we learn from our teachers is ours to keep. It can benefit us for a lifetime and it can never be taken away.

Having a good teacher also motivates us to continue to improve, whether we practise alone or with a group. Practising regularly develops strong internal stability and strength, leading to more vitality, better focused energy and a clearer mind.[31]

Longevity through qi exercises

Chinese books are full of stories of people who restored their health with Chinese exercises. One tells of a Chinese man who came from a poor family. He had to sell vegetables at the local fair from a young age and he carried them on a pole that rested on his shoulders. By the time he was 12 he had developed a hunched back and was nicknamed 'the hunchbacked vegetable boy'. He later learned Chinese boxing – a martial art where concentration on the *dantien* is practised. He eventually straightened his back. He was still strong and robust at 100 and taught other children Chinese boxing throughout his life.[32]

In another story a doctor became weakened when he developed tuberculosis at the age of 48. He practised *qigong* under a famous teacher. By learning *qigong* his lung trouble cleared without any treatment and he subsequently became a practicitioner of Chinese medicine and worked until he was nearly 100 years old.[33]

Action Box

Finding a teacher

The best way to find a good teacher is by word of mouth. Talk to existing learners and find out about the benefits they reap from their practice. Before joining a class you might want to talk to the teacher to discuss the type of *qigong* practice she or he teaches.

67 A simple self-exercise more effective than massage

This simple patting exercise can have profound effects. It is good for strengthening the tendons, bones and muscles, improving the circulation and enhancing the functioning of the internal organs. After patting the body we will feel wide awake, ready for action, clear-headed and our spirits will be lifted. Patting is said to be more effective than massage performed by other people. The whole body is lightly patted with either palms or fists, in eight main areas (see Figure 11).

Stand with the feet shoulder-width apart and relax the whole body. Make sure that your knees are slightly bent and your feet are facing forwards. Breathe naturally as you do the exercise.

Pat the head
Pat both sides of the head with the palms or fists from the front of the head to the back. Pat to and fro for about 20 times.

Pat the arms
Pat up and down the front, back and sides of the left arm with the right palm or fist 10 times on each side. Then pat the right arm with the left palm or fist in the same way.

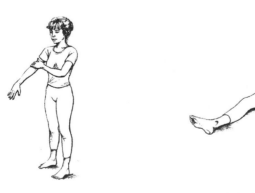

Figure 11. Patting the arms and the legs.

Pat the shoulders

Pat the left shoulder with the right palm or fist and the right shoulder with the left palm or fist. Pat them alternatively for 10 times each.

Pat the back

Pat up and down the right side of the lower back with the left palm or fist, then the left side of the lower back with the right palm or fist, for 20 times each side.

Pat the chest

Pat the left and right sides of the chest with the opposite palm or fist alternately. Pat from the top to the bottom then the bottom to the top for 20 times on each side.

Pat the waist and abdomen

Taking the waist as an axis turn the upper body to the left then to the right. As you turn, pat the left side of the waist with the right palm or fist and the right side of the waist with the left palm or fist. Pat from top to bottom and move from the inside of the waist and abdomen outwards. Pat 20 times on each side.

Pat the buttocks

Pat the left buttocks with the left palm or fist and the right buttock with the right palm or fist. Pat 20 times on each side.

Pat the legs

Sit on the floor with legs outstretched and knees bent up. Pat up and down the front, back and sides of the legs with both hands, from the top of the leg downwards, for 40 times each side.

Action Box

A summary of the patting self-exercise:

- Pat the head.
- Pat the arms.
- Pat the shoulders.
- Pat the back.
- Pat the chest.
- Pat the waist and abdomen.
- Pat the buttocks.
- Pat the legs.

68 Use Chinese metal balls as a simple longevity tool

Chinese 'metal' balls are easily available from many Chinese shops. They have been used since the Ming dynasty (1368–1644 CE) to strengthen the *qi* and the constitution.

The use of these balls is based on the theory of traditional Chinese medicine. Acupuncture channels circulate *qi* throughout the body and the pathways travel around the body, forming a circuit. The *qi* can easily be massaged at the extremities, especially in the hands. Moving the balls activates the energy channels and this in turn strengthens the connected Organs.

By circulating the balls all the vital Organs can be strengthened. The brain can also be strengthened as it connects to the *qi* pathways in the hands. This keeps the memory strong and the brain clear and active. Using the balls encourages longevity and is easy to do while sitting watching TV, listening to music or reading.

Action Box

To use Chinese metal balls:

- Hold two balls on one palm and move them in a circular direction using an opening and closing motion of the fingers.
- At first this may seem awkward and the movement will be uneven. In time, however, it will become increasingly smooth.
- Once the movement is smooth in one direction learn to turn them in the opposite direction. This too will be awkward at first and will gradually become smoother in time.
- Circulate the balls with both hands equally and do this for at least five minutes a day.
- Start with smaller balls, and for an additional challenge either use larger balls or use more balls in the palm of one hand.
- Increase your ability slowly and surely – don't expect to become an expert without practice!

6 Secrets to Protect Ourselves from the Environment

How the weather affects our health

I'm like everyone else who was brought up in Britain. One of my first topics of conversation is the weather. Many of us do it without thinking. We meet and comment on the cold by pulling ourselves in and wrapping our arms around ourselves. Or the damp – it's so muggy and heavy and d-u-l-l. Let's hope it brightens up soon. And the wind – it really gets to you, doesn't it? It penetrates. It makes it feel even colder. Then at last the sun shines. We love it and the whole country brightens up and we all chat to each other and become friendlier. But after a while we start to moan. It's really too hot and it's humid too. I can't bear it any longer – too much heat!

The weather is a part of our everyday lives. Well, there's so much weather for us British people to deal with! It affects us all the time. We get 'under the weather'. We're often not conscious of the effect it's having but we're experiencing it in our body.

When I first learnt Chinese medicine it put into words what I'd unconsciously known about the climate:

- Damp makes us feel heavy and sluggish.

- Cold slows us down and makes us contract inside.

- Wind drives in other climatic factors with what we now call the 'wind-chill factor'.

- We become more expansive in the heat – but if we get too much of it or if it's damp and hot, it makes us feel tired and sluggish.

In the past, all cultures were aware of the weather's effect on their health. Chinese medicine has retained this knowledge and it has been passed down through generations. In the West this has mostly been lost. This is especially in the years since the Second World War when this wisdom, often found in 'old wives' tales', has been discarded.

I was born just after the war and I learnt various old wives' tales from my parents. 'Don't sleep with wet hair', 'wrap up against the cold', 'avoid sitting in a draught', 'wear warm slippers'. When I was young these seemed to be pointless and I ignored them. When I learnt Chinese medicine I realized that they were in fact wise sayings. The effects of wind, cold, damp, dryness and heat are known to Chinese medicine as the climatic or 'external' causes of disease.

We are all affected by at least one climate. Invariably in the UK either the cold or the damp affects the largest number of people. This is closely followed by the wind and heat. Not surprisingly in such a damp country, very few are affected by excess dryness – although in Arizona or the Sahara it is different.

These external climatic conditions can have as big an impact on our health as our emotions and we can become healthier if we learn to protect ourselves from them. In this chapter we'll discuss some simple lifestyle changes that will ensure better health if we heed them. Meanwhile you might think about which climatic conditions affect you the most and how you protect yourself from them.

69 Take extra care when there's a cold snap

When we're cold our body reacts. We slow down. We shiver, trying to warm ourselves up. Our body contracts to protect us. We are most affected by the cold in three circumstances:

- If there is a 'cold snap', for example, an unexpected plunge in temperature in the middle of milder weather.

- When the cold is prolonged, for example in a long cold winter.

- If we are particularly frail – then we may be more susceptible to the cold.

It may surprise you to know that the cold is responsible for more deaths and other health disorders than most other weather conditions. We might think that in the 21st century, when we have warm homes, indoor toilets and warm clothes, it would no longer be a problem. Although the elderly, children and sick people are most affected by the cold, we are all susceptible and many illnesses are due to the cold.

The winter of 1963 was one of the coldest in Europe since the beginning of the 20th century. In that year the mortality of people over 60 years old increased by 15.7% compared with the previous winter. The cold weather puts extra stress on the organs of those who are already ill. There are more strokes, heart attacks and respiratory infections in the winter. Even the incidence of death from illnesses such as cirrhosis of the liver, diabetes and cancer is increased. Old and frail people are the most susceptible to cold and other climatic conditions as their *qi* is weaker.[1]

Cold affects some people more than others. If you're always sitting close to fires and radiators and love holidays in sunny climates you probably have a greater tendency to be affected by it.

If you are affected by the cold it can directly affect your health. One of my colleagues hates the cold weather. If her feet get too cold or she gets chilled, she can end up 'catching a chill'.

Cold can affect those who are vulnerable to it, but can also affect anyone who is unavoidably caught in it for any length of time. One patient came to me having got chilled waiting in the cold for a friend. She'd tried to keep warm by walking around but she still got cold. The next day she had diarrhoea. She'd got chilled in her stomach from the cold and damp and the loose bowels were her body's reaction.

Some time ago a politician in England advised old people to wear long johns and woolly hats when it was cold. She was laughed at for her old-fashioned and rather tactless advice – people thought she was trying to avoid giving much-needed funding to the elderly. Leaving aside the politics and the context in which the advice was given, her advice was in fact very sound. Long johns and hats are a sensible choice for many of us.

Action Box

These ways of protecting yourself from the cold might seem obvious but affect our health if ignored:

- **Wear layers rather than just one thick fabric**. The layers trap warmth and protect the body better than only one thickness. Include thermal vests and long underwear, long coats past the knee and more than one jumper.
- **Wear gloves and hats as well as warm shoes and socks**. Those old wives' tales that tell us to wear a hat when it's cold and not to walk around without shoes on give us really sensible advice. Heat is easily lost from the extremities.
- **Heat your environment adequately**. Try to keep at least one room well heated. Living in a cold house can not only make us ill but we can also become depressed.
- **Be aware of your constitution**. If you are a naturally chilly person, cold will have a greater effect than if you are more warm-blooded. Older people are particularly vulnerable to the cold.
- **Be aware of the seasons**. When the weather is hot we can wear fewer clothes, swim in cold water or eat colder food – but not in the cold winter.

70 Your pain might be caused by cold!

In the cold of wintertime nature slows down and everything contracts. It is the time of conservation and storage. But the cold can also be ruthless. When we are slightly cold, we feel chilled and we shiver; during extreme cold our body contracts against it. If the cold is continuous or intense we contract even more, resulting in extreme pain.

We have all experienced the effects of cold. For example, on a snowy day if you hold a handful of snow, your fingers will start to hurt. If you eat ice cream too quickly it can get stuck in your gullet, causing pain until it passes into your stomach. On a cold day your ears might be painful if they are not protected. These symptoms are all due to the tissues contracting.

The pain from cold is sharp and intense. Cold can be the cause of a range of pains, such as period pains, joint pains, back pain, some headaches or abdominal pains – in fact, any sharp, intense and 'biting' pain. And of course these pains are always relieved to some degree by heat.

Some (not all) period pains can be caused by the cold. At one time young girls were made to play sports outdoors in the middle of winter – wearing shorts. This was seen as 'healthy'! For some this was the cause of period pains that plagued them through to adulthood. Others say that swimming in cold water and getting chilled could have been the initial cause of their period pains; or even making love during a period, a time when the uterus is particularly vulnerable to cold.

Joint pains have many causes. A friend of mine, when she was a child, often scrubbed celery in freezing water in her father's greengrocers. Years later she got very painful arthritis in her fingers, which had never recovered. Back pain can be caused by a change in temperature. For example, a man digging his garden may take his shirt off as he works in the heat. His pores open as he sweats. Then the sun goes in and he gets chilled. The pores close. The next day he has a backache caused by the trapped cold. He doesn't connect it and doesn't know why he's in pain.

Protecting ourselves from these cold conditions can save ourselves a lifetime of pain. Once we have long-term pain caused by cold, putting heat on the area is often not enough. Acupuncture or another Chinese medicine may be needed to cure the condition. Better to protect ourselves now!

> ### Action Box
>
> To avoid pain, protect yourself from cold:
>
> - Notice any sharp pains you feel when you are out in cold weather. It is a sign that an area is affected by the cold – so cover up. This can be painful ears, hands, feet or head.
> - If you do get stomach pains from the cold, immediately put something warm on the area, such as a hot water bottle.

Also take note of the suggestions in Secret 69.

 # 71 Cold can cause infertility and other lower-body symptoms

There are three main Organs where Chinese medicine says cold can enter the body. They are the stomach, the lower abdomen and the uterus.

Cold can cause many symptoms in the lower body, often without our realizing it. Some we've already discussed such as period pains, abdominal pains and back pain. Others include infertility and scanty periods, stomach upsets, diarrhoea, cold feet and other circulation problems, watery discharges or profuse urination.

Cold, infertility and other effects on the uterus

You may be surprised to know that, according to Chinese medicine, cold in the uterus is one of the most common causes of infertility. By warming and moving the *qi* in the abdomen, acupuncture can often help. Much better, though, is to prevent this from happening. Let's look at some of the underlying causes.

During the time women are menstruating Chinese medicine practitioners have noted that our uterus is more vulnerable to the effects of cold. Two famous old wives' tales are, 'Don't make love during your period' and 'Don't swim during your period'. Since the coming of tampons we may have thrown this second piece of sound advice to the wind (or maybe we should say to the cold as well!).

Another saying is, 'Don't sit on stone steps', and this would now include metal seats –a relatively recent innovation. A patient commented on the metal seats now found in railway stations. 'We used to have such lovely wooden seats and they were warm and easy to sit on if you were tired. I notice that within a short time of sitting on metal ones I feel uncomfortable and disturbed as the cold is coming up into my abdomen.'

If we don't cover our feet the cold can travel up the legs to the uterus. I have a patient who now has two children. She couldn't conceive for many years because of cold in the uterus. She had been walking around on stone floors without shoes, oblivious to consequences. She became pregnant only when she started wearing slippers!

Cold and the lower abdomen and stomach

I cringe inside when I see teenagers leaving their bellies uncovered. Fashionable it may be but healthy it isn't. They may not connect their health problems with the way they dress.

An old Chinese saying is that 'the digestive organs like warmth'. When we leave our abdomen exposed to the cold it can affect our stomach and intestines, causing vomiting, loose bowels and abdominal pain. It can also slow down our metabolism and be a reason for putting on weight.

Eating too much cold food may also affect our stomach and lower abdomen. This includes raw food, ice cream and iced drinks as well as foods whose 'nature' is cold, such as tofu and other soya products. Cold foods are best eaten along with something warming to counteract the cold. Nourishing soups or other warm food, especially in the winter, can prevent many digestive and bowel problems due to cold. These are discussed in greater depth in Chapter 3.

> ### Action Box
>
> Here are some other ways you can protect your lower body from the cold:
>
> - Avoid cold metal seats or stone steps. Protect yourself by sitting on a newspaper or magazine or even carrying a blow-up cushion. It may be better to stand if there is nothing else available. This especially applies to people who have sensitivity to cold including women who have a tendency to get period pains from cold in the uterus.
> - Avoid leaving the abdomen uncovered even if it is fashionable to do so. Even in mild weather cold can 'invade' the abdomen or back causing stomach, bowel, or back problems or even infertility or period pains.
> - Take care with cold food (see pages 38 and 55). It can cause stomach pain, loose bowels and other abdominal symptoms, especially if eaten in vast quantities or if you have a tendency to feel the cold. When it's cold it's important to eat hotter food and keep warm.
> - Protect yourself so that cold doesn't travel up your legs to your abdomen. Wear slippers and keep your feet warm.
> - Cover your legs in the cold. Women who wear miniskirts in the cold tend to accumulate subcutaneous fat on their thighs to protect them. Wearing thicker tights or even two layers of tights will prevent this – and ensure you don't put weight on your legs.

Also note the other suggestions in Secrets 69 and 70 above.

72 A well-kept secret – the effects of 'wind'

In some situations the wind may have an impact on our wellbeing. Unlike cold, wind is not commonly described in the West in relation to our health. In spite of this many people know that wind affects them.

How severe windy weather affects our health has been well documented in many countries. Nations in Central Europe describe *fohn* winds. North Americans describe *chinook* and *santa ana* winds. Israelis know when the *sharav* blows. Australians are aware of Easterlies, Westerlies or Northerlies. These winds are all said to cause problems, which vary from headaches and migraines to an increased incidence of accident, crime and suicide rates.[2]

Chinese medicine uses the term 'wind' as a metaphor. Wind in the body is like wind in nature. Any conditions that arise suddenly, come and go rapidly and go through many swift changes are 'wind'. Most conditions of wind are also located in the top, outer surface part of the body.

In Chinese medicine wind is termed 'the spearhead of disease'. According to one famous Chinese saying: 'Wind is the chief of the 100 diseases and it makes other climatic causes penetrate.' Wind can be the means by which cold, heat, damp and dryness are driven into the body.

We can compare this with the 'wind-chill factor' that we often hear about on weather forecasts. Wind-chill describes how a strong wind exaggerates our experience of cold. Put another way, we could say that the higher the wind-chill factor, the more cold is being driven into the body. Because wind can drive in other diseases, many Chinese medicine texts suggest that we avoid exercising in the wind. We can take note of ways suggested in Secret 69 to avoid cold, such as wearing gloves, hats and coats.

There are two main ways in which we can be affected by wind: being caught in windy conditions, and sudden weather changes.

'Windy' conditions

Windy conditions can mean anything from a mild breeze to a storm. Obviously the effects of a storm such as a gale, hurricane, typhoon or tornado are likely to be greater than those of a breeze.

Another 'wind' condition is a draught. When a patient came to me recently with a stiff neck it didn't take me long to discover why. The previous day she had driven with the window open to keep her cool. The 'wind' had penetrated her neck. Now she couldn't move her head from side to side. She hadn't realized that this 'wind' had brought it on overnight.

Fortunately it took only one acupuncture treatment to free her neck, but she could have prevented this debilitating condition if she'd remembered that we should avoid draughts and cover our neck in the wind.

You may be surprised to know that we can be affected by 'wind' that is artificial. The breeze created by a fan or from air conditioning in homes, cars or buildings can be just as debilitating if we are susceptible. I remember being at a conference when the room was too hot. The organizers used a high-speed fan that blasted out air like a gale-force wind to cool the participants down. Subsequently many people in the room became ill with colds and influenza. Again this would have been unnecessary if people had realized the potential effects of this 'draught'.

Sudden weather changes

A sudden change can mean any unseasonal change in the weather. How many of us have gone abroad to somewhere warm in winter and caught a cold as soon as we came home? This is a common situation we don't think much about. The changes in temperature when we move in and out of shops and other centrally heated or air-conditioned buildings can also have an effect. My mother always used to tell me to put on or take off extra clothes when going from warm to cold environments. Another helpful piece of advice was to wrap up warmly when travelling home from abroad for when the temperature drops.

Action Box

Ensure that you are protected from wind:

- Take care in changing temperatures. Put on or take off clothes. This is especially necessary if you are returning from warm holidays abroad to a cold climate or when moving in and out of heated shops in cold weather.
- Avoid draughts or wind created by fans and air conditioning of any kind. Especially avoid sleeping in a draught or sitting or standing directly in front of a fan. Take care to wear enough clothes to protect yourself when you are in air-conditioned environments.

73 How to prevent colds, flu and other acute problems

Wind and the common cold

Chinese medicine describes 'wind' as rapidly changing symptoms that arise suddenly and are close to the top of the body. So it's not surprising that a common cold is described as 'an attack of wind'. For example, this is how one patient described his cold. 'It came on overnight when I woke with a sore throat. The next day my nose was running, my jaw ached, my eyes hurt and I felt extremely tired and shivery. Two days later all my symptoms had gone during the day, yet I still woke up coughing at night. Five days later it had gone completely.'

A mixture of elements causes most acute infections, with wind as a 'spearhead' driving in another climatic cause. Because the above patient was chilled as well as having fast-changing symptoms, his diagnosis was 'wind and cold'. Infections that involve a high temperature or a red sore throat would be 'wind and heat'.

But you might ask – don't infections come from germs? The answer is 'yes'. Chinese doctors discovered that droplet infection could cause colds as far back as the Qing dynasty around 1700.[3] These doctors realized that knowing about germs did not protect us from illness – there will always be germs around that we can 'catch'. What protects us from infections is keeping our surface *qi* strong. This is the equivalent to keeping our immune system strong. When we are trying to adjust to changes in climate or other causes of 'wind', our immune system is weakened and we are more vulnerable to 'catching' infections.

Wind and other acute symptoms

Other symptoms of wind could be joint pains that move around or come and go (as opposed to pain from cold which is a contracting pain). Symptoms that come on suddenly such as neck pain, facial paralysis, severe dizziness or acute headaches can also be due to wind.

Research carried out as far back as the late 1950s provided some insight into the effects of wind or changes in the weather on our health. It established that many rheumatic attacks that were severe enough for a person to stop work were often related to changes in the weather. Over a period of two years researchers followed a group of 35 outpatients with rheumatic symptoms. One of their findings was: 'The most harmful meteorological events are a sudden drop in temperature, strong winds and the influx of polar air masses.'[4]

Another researcher observed that all forms of rheumatic disease are more common in Turkey than in many other countries. In Turkey, summers are very hot and winters very cold. People in the capital, Ankara, where temperatures are extreme are especially susceptible. In comparison, the incidence of rheumatic problems is low in areas around the equator. Here the heat is constant and there is little difference between summer and winter.[5]

In reality we rarely know the actual events that led up to us 'catching' a cold or other acute conditions. Sometimes we don't remember getting chilled, being caught in windy conditions or being affected by weather changes. It doesn't matter. If we protect ourselves from these climatic conditions we will keep healthier and be less susceptible to acute symptoms. In Chinese medicine having rapidly changing symptoms that are in the upper part of the body and which move around are enough to make the diagnosis of 'an attack of wind'.

Action Box

Here are some other ways that we can protect ourselves from wind.

- Wear a scarf to protect your neck and head in the wind to prevent colds, flu and stiff necks.
- Wind and cold can easily combine, so any of the suggestions for protecting ourselves from cold also apply to some extent to protection from the wind. Wearing gloves, hats and warm footwear are all important steps in protecting ourselves from infections.
- Avoid exercising in the wind. This is important if you become hot when exercising and your pores open. The wind can easily 'invade' through the pores, making us susceptible to catching infections.

- Be aware that wind can also affect the joints if they are not protected. Pain caused by wind tends to come and go and move from place to place.
- If you are feeling tired, shocked, emotionally upset or are 'under the weather' in any way, be extra vigilant about protecting yourself from wind. Your immune system may be weakened, making you more susceptible.

Also note other suggestions in Secret 72.

74 Tired all the time? 'Damp' could be the cause

The feeling of being tired all the time is endemic in many Western countries. Reasons for this include overwork, poor diet and not enough sleep. One other reason is little known in the West. Tiredness can also be caused by dampness.

Chinese medicine describes dampness as sticky, heavy and lingering – all things we feel when the weather is damp.

Some people are more vulnerable to dampness than others. If you are vulnerable you may feel extremely lethargic – especially on very dull, damp or humid days. You may also feel heavy-limbed, stiff, achy and a bit depressed. Some people feel better as soon as the day brightens up. For others it takes longer and they only feel better when out of the damp for some time.

Living in a damp country can be enough to affect our susceptibility to some degree. Britain is a very damp country, with Wales and other areas in the west being particularly problematic.

Other symptoms of damp

If you dislike damp weather, this may indicate that you are vulnerable to its effects. In general, the weather we are most sensitive to has the most negative effect on our health. One patient who dislikes damp weather describes going outside and feeling the wet air penetrate. 'I feel powerless to keep it out.' His immediate response is that he wants to get away from it – it slows him down and makes him feel exhausted. The dehumidifiers in his house ease some of the detrimental effects.

Some people feel their joints become achy when the weather is damp. This signals that damp has penetrated them. We all know people who can literally predict damp weather as they feel it in their joints. My granny always knew damp weather was on its way as she felt it in her knees.

Another common symptom of damp is a muzzy head. One patient who got soaked in the rain said she couldn't think for a while and it felt as if she had a 'damp' brain, 'like cotton wool was in there'.

The lethargy that comes from damp is often described by people as a heavy feeling combined with a desire to lie down a lot. One of my patients who was affected by damp had a favourite saying: 'Why stand when you can sit and why sit if you can lie down.'

Other symptoms of damp include feeling heavy-limbed, a lack of concentration, a stuffy feeling in the chest or abdomen, oozing discharges or loose stools. The movement of damp is downwards and because it is heavy and lingering it often affects the lower body. This is in contrast to wind that travels upwards, changes quickly and is easier to move. Damp tends to be the hardest climatic cause of disease to clear from our system. If you get that tired-all-the-time feeling or other symptoms of damp, Secret 75 will suggest ways of clearing it.

Action Box

If you feel lethargic, tired and heavy and this gets worse on damp or humid days, be aware that it might be due to dampness. Other symptoms are a muzzy head, achy limbs, lack of concentration, a stuffy feeling in the chest or abdomen, oozing discharges or loose stools. Protect yourself from these damp-forming situations by noting the list in the action box of the next secret.

75 Protect yourself from the effects of damp

As well as living in a damp country or environment we can be affected by other damp conditions such as:

- frequently being in or near water

- living in a damp house

- wearing damp clothes

- sitting on damp grass

- not drying ourselves properly.

Frequently being in or near water or living in a damp house

One of my patients used to work on a trout farm that was situated at the bottom of a valley and on top of a spring – a very damp environment! He described feeling so totally lethargic that he would lie around doing nothing most of the time. 'No one used to talk to me for one and a half hours after I got up as I was so obnoxious and I could only do routine things.' He told me this after it had become a thing of the past. Once he moved away from this environment he got much better – although he remained slightly vulnerable to the damp weather.

If you live near or by water, rivers, the sea, lakes or live near marshy land, you should be careful to protect yourself from the effects of dampness. Also if you live on a boat or in places that 'catch' the damp, such as valleys or low-lying land. If you live in a damp environment and are particularly susceptible, a dehumidifier may help or a good damp-proof course in your house. Acupuncture or herbs may also help to clear the effects of dampness. For really susceptible people the only solution could be to move to a drier environment.

Other causes of dampness

Our grannies in their wisdom would always insist on putting their clothes in an airing cupboard before wearing them. This removed any remaining dampness and prevented rheumatic problems. They would also say that you should always change out of wet clothes.

If your clothes are damp because you've been sweating make sure you change them – but not until you have finished sweating. If you change your clothes while still sweating your pores will be open. In this case damp and cold can easily get in and you can catch a chill or develop joint problems.

Another saying suggests that you shouldn't sit around on wet grass. A colleague and her friends went rowing on a canal in Amsterdam. After the strenuous activity she lay down on the grass to rest. Soon afterwards she flew home and the next day woke up unable to move. The grass had been damp and it had penetrated the muscles in her back, causing them to seize up. An acupuncturist used a 'cupping' treatment and removed the damp and she could move again. She could have avoided the problem by not having laid down on the wet grass, or to have lain on a blanket, but sometimes we only learn from experience.

Drying ourselves properly

Other old wives' tales tell us to dry ourselves thoroughly after bathing, not to go out with wet hair, and not to go to sleep with wet hair. A friend who is now a practitioner told me that when she was young she knew she should not to go out with wet hair. She hit on a good idea when she was in her teens. She would wash her hair at night, place a towel on her pillow and in the morning – wonderful – she had dry hair. She didn't have to go out with wet hair! Every year she got bronchitis but never connected it with what she was doing – until she learnt Chinese medicine when she was 31. She stopped this bad habit and never had bronchitis again and is now careful with her health in every way.

If we go out or sleep with wet hair we can become more vulnerable to wind and cold as well as damp and can easily get coughs, colds and chest infections.

Diet and damp

Some foods are said to be more phlegm and damp-forming than others. These tend to be 'sticky' foods such as excess dairy produce, bananas, peanuts and greasy food. Eating too much of these foods will increase the amount of damp in our body. For more on damp-forming foods, turn to pages 40–41.

Action Box

The following are reminders of a few ways to protect yourself from damp:

- Buy a dehumidifier to dry out your house if it is damp.
- A good damp-proof course may prevent damp from penetrating into your home.
- Avoid getting chest conditions by drying your hair before going out and never sleeping with wet hair.
- Keep your body dry and protected from damp. Dry yourself thoroughly after swimming or bathing. Wear dry clothes and do not sit in damp places.
- If your clothes are damp because you've been sweating, change them after you've finished sweating.
- If you are vulnerable to damp, be careful about the food you eat and avoid the damp-forming foods mentioned on pages 40–41.

76 Dryness – of course it dries you up!

Dryness as a cause of disease is seen less in many parts of the West than cold, wind and damp. This doesn't mean that we aren't affected by it.

The main symptoms of dryness are, not surprisingly, dry symptoms – a dry nose, dry throat, dry eyes, dry mouth, dry skin or a dry cough with little sputum.

Who is affected by dryness?

Those typically affected are people who work in dry, centrally heated environments or live in very dry houses. The atmosphere in aeroplanes can also be very dry and drinking lots of water can prevent us from dehydrating.

Just as Britain is a damp country, other countries can be very dry. Once on a trip to China many of my friends became ill. One of them told me: 'I remember stepping outside in Beijing and breathing in. I had the extraordinary feeling of the cold and dryness going through my nose and deep into my lungs.' A few days later it turned into an infection, which she experienced as a dryness in her lungs and an aching feeling in her chest. She also had a hacking cough but no matter how much she coughed she just couldn't produce anything. She had what Chinese medicine calls 'Lung dryness'.

Action Box

Living and working in a dry environment can be very debilitating and leave us exposed to getting symptoms of dryness. Here are some simple means of combating dryness:

- Place a bowl of water in the room. Some people hang containers of water from a radiator.
- A more sophisticated method of dealing with dryness is to get a humidifier.
- If you are suffering from a dry cough or infection, breathing in steam from a bowl of hot water or breathing vapour into the lungs will help to bring moisture to the throat and chest. Vaporizers can be brought from old-fashioned chemists and some health-food shops.
- The atmosphere of a plane can be very drying. When flying drink lots of water to make sure you don't dehydrate.

 Know how to beat the heat

Heat can heal or it can burn you up. After a long, cold winter the sun brings us out of our houses and we become more active and sociable. Our bodies are better equipped to deal with heat than with cold. When we are warm, the blood vessels at skin level dilate and allow the heat to escape. We also perspire. As the perspiration evaporates we cool down.

If, however, we are exposed to the heat for long periods we may become ill. People who work in hot laundries or bakeries can suffer the impact of heat as well as those who are affected by the sun.

The effects of the sun

Heat can injure and kill. In 1996 Pakistan and India experienced temperatures of up to 49 degrees Celsius in the shade. The Indian press reported a death toll of 2,500 but acknowledged that the numbers were probably higher. In colder climates such as Britain or the Netherlands we can take less heat. If the temperature rises sharply above 25 degrees, the death rate rises.[6]

Until the 1920s people in the West didn't sunbathe much. It was fashionable to remain pale and stay in the shade. Then Coco Chanel of the Chanel fashion house went on a cruise and came back with a suntan. A new craze for suntans was born and everyone wanted one. All of us sun-worshippers who once lay in the sun for hours now know that we need to take extra care to avoid its worst effects. Those who live in sunny climates know to treat the sun with respect by not overexposing themselves to it.

Signs and symptoms of heat exhaustion

Symptoms of prolonged exposure are irritability, high fever, cramps, rapid breathing and palpitations. If exposure continues or is extreme it will become serious. Our temperature rises and we get dehydrated. Later we can go into shock and heart failure.

Since the discovery of holes in the ozone layer and the increase in the incidence of skin cancer, ways of protecting ourselves from the heat and sun are well documented. Most people who holiday frequently or live in hot countries are well aware of the effects of the sun.

Action Box

Ways to protect yourself from the heat:

- Do not stay out in the sun for long periods. Find a shady spot whenever possible.
- Make sure you drink enough liquids so that you don't dehydrate. Thirst is the first sign of dehydration in most people.
- If you like to sunbathe build up slowly and don't – like mad dogs and Englishmen – stay out in the midday sun.
- Protect your skin with high-factor sun creams that are made from natural ingredients. Sunburnt skin prevents us cooling down easily.
- Take regular cool showers if you are too hot.
- Don't do strenuous activity in the sun.
- Diet can also generate heat in the body. Heating foods include meats such as lamb and beef and hot curries. For more on heating food see page 56.
- Many people living in hot countries take a short siesta after their lunch. They know that it's best to avoid going out in the sun when it's at its hottest. After their siesta they wake up refreshed and can enjoy themselves well into the evening.
- People in hot countries often wear clothes that protect them from the sun. A shirt or blouse with sleeves is a better choice than a sleeveless top as this protects the shoulders. Wear a wide-brimmed hat to protect the skin on the face and head. Light-coloured clothes reflect radiation.
- Be aware that nothing ages your skin faster than too much sun, which dries up the skin on the face.
- Hot drinks may cool you down better than cold drinks. Green tea, for instance, is cooling in nature and can be sipped slowly.

Other effects of heat

External heat can make us ill but heat can also be generated internally. Chinese medicine notes that overwork or unresolved emotions can generate heat in our systems. During menopause many women get hot flushes. This heat is internally generated. It is due to the decline of the moistening and cooling *yin* aspects of the body at this time of life. For more on menopause and overworking, turn to Chapter 5 on work, rest and exercise. For lifestyle advice about hot flushes, see page 221, and for more on the emotions see Chapter 4.

78 Flow with the seasons to stay healthy

Some countries have huge seasonal variations in temperature while others have less changeable climates. We can adjust our lifestyle as the seasons vary. If we look at animals we notice that they change from season to season.

Animals adapt to winter temperatures by growing thick protective coats or hibernating. In a similar way we need to wear thicker clothes at this time of year. The Chinese note that in winter, when it is darker and colder, we should go to bed earlier, get up later and be less active.

In summer the animals lose their winter coats and are at their most energetic. In general we too are more active in summer and can go to bed later and rise earlier.

In spring the climate is more changeable and we can protect ourselves against wind and rain. An old saying states: 'Ne'er cast a clout till May is out.' This means don't cast off your warm clothes until May has gone. In autumn, of course, we should take care to add more layers of clothes as the weather gets colder.

We are all affected by the elements, but the healthier we are, the fewer negative effects we experience. Balancing our diet, emotions, work, rest and exercise as well as looking after our constitution can help us to achieve good health.

Food and water are becoming increasingly polluted (in Chapter 3 we discussed the purity of our food). The air is also polluted by traffic fumes, especially in urban areas. Spending more time in an environment that has clean air can be very restorative to our health. This can just be a walk in the countryside or by a river. Sadly the days are long gone when doctors sent their patients to the seaside to convalesce or when patients with tuberculosis were sent to the mountains to breathe fresh air. A healthy atmosphere and restful conditions are very healing.

Action Box

We can adjust to the seasons to remain healthy. In spring and summer we are more active, wear fewer clothes, eat cooler or neutral food, go to bed later and rise earlier. In autumn and winter we can wear clothing to protect ourselves from the cold, slow down and do less, eat more warm food, go to bed later and rise later to conserve energy.

7 Secrets of Making Lifestyle Changes

Get ready to make lifestyle changes that stick!

Below are some useful secrets that will enable you to make long-lasting and effective lifestyle improvements. They are written in the spirit of Chinese medicine, which suggests we make lifestyle adjustments in a balanced and harmonious way. Changing our lifestyle slowly, with sensitivity and without forcing things, enables us to make lifestyle changes that *really* stick!

79 Four important stages of integrating lifestyle changes

There are four main stages to go through before a lifestyle adjustment is fully integrated into your life. You'll move through some of these stages very quickly. Others might take longer. The stages are:

1. intention
2. preparation
3. action
4. completion and integration.

People who don't successfully make a change or who keep falling back usually haven't gone through all these steps – so it's best to take note of them all – especially when you're making major lifestyle alterations. This secret will take you through these four stages in detail.

1. Refine your intention

The first stage of changing your lifestyle is to have the *intention* to do it. It can take either a long time or a short time to decide to do something – no hurry. Weigh it up. Check it out – is this right for you? Don't pick too much to do. Doing too much can be overwhelming.

Some people stay at this stage for a few hours, some a few months. Others take many years! We *intend* to eat more healthily. We *intend* to go to bed earlier. We *intend* to start exercising – but we haven't started the process of making the change. If you know what you intend to do but can't put it into action you may need ask yourself: 'What's stopping me from making this improvement?'

Action Box
Know what's stopping you

If you know what you intend to do but can't put it into action, here are some things to consider:

- Are you well motivated to do it? Have you got a *carrot* – or something attracting you, as well as a *stick* – something you don't want to happen if you don't change?
- Is what you intend to do rather vague – do you need a more *specific plan*?
- Are you trying to change too much – do you need to take *smaller steps*?
- Is this improvement right for you – should you consider *choosing something else*?
- Do you think you should be perfect – do you need to *loosen up*?
- Are you ready to make the improvement – is the *timing* right?
- Is it what *you* want to do – is *someone else pushing you*?

2. Prepare to change your lifestyle

You may have decided on the change you want to make but are wondering *how* to do it. It is often useful to have someone to discuss this with – a health professional, a friend or a partner. If you're giving up some food, have you found a substitute? (See page 61 for a list of common food substitutes.) If you're looking at emotional issues do you need more of a support system? If you're changing the way you're exercising, do you need to practise with a group?

Action Box
Preparing your plan

Once you have a plan, write down:

- What you intend to do.
- How you intend to do it.
- Your start date.
- A date at which you will assess the impact of the change.

You may want to stick your plan to the fridge door or put it in a prominent position and refer back to it if you feel your resolve waning. *Putting it in writing helps you to stay committed.* Check inside yourself – are you completely ready? You may find that telling others can increase the level of your commitment. If you've planned well and you know you are ready, once your start date arrives you'll easily put it into action.

---

3. Put your lifestyle plan into action

You've made your plan – this first stage of this step is easy – just jump into it!

After your initial enthusiasm, however, the going can become more difficult. Some people go through a wobbly stage. This is quite normal if you're making a major lifestyle change. If you get to the wobbly stage feel really pleased! You're in 'transition' and have nearly succeeded in making a long-term adjustment.

You can compare this with giving birth. Anyone who has been through childbirth knows about that important stage called 'transition'. At this stage the would-be mother who has endured contractions and pain but is getting through, suddenly wants to give up and thinks she can't go through with it – she decides she doesn't

171

want to give birth at all! Those who are in the know reassure her at this stage. They know it is a sign that the baby is about to be born! It only lasts a short time and the baby begins to arrive.

If you want to give up on the planned adjustment, this means you've nearly competed making the change! Stay with it.

Action Box
Be prepared for the wobbly stage!

Some lifestyle adjustments take staying power. In general the better prepared you are the more likely you are to keep going at exercising, writing your journal, keeping up the dietary change or whatever else you plan. So it is not always best to move to this stage *too* quickly.

4. Completion and integration – make a new adjustment into a regular habit

Once you have completed making a lifestyle change you're working towards making it a regular habit. Before getting to this stage you may have gone through some slight struggles in ensuring you keep your resolve. The completion stage is much easier.

Action Box
Remember – it takes a month to change a habit!

The main thing to remember from when you start improving your lifestyle is that Chinese wisdom tells us *it takes at least a month to change a habit.* After about a month from when you began and the change will be more or less in place.

Remembering that it takes a month can help us to go through any discomfort we might encounter early on. We can bear in mind that difficulties will ease after the first month – following this the adjustments will internalize and become a part of our normal lifestyle.

When a lifestyle change is fully integrated into your life it is so much a part of your routine that you don't even have to think about doing it. In fact, if you don't do it for some reason you miss it!

80 Find ways to become motivated

We need to feel well motivated in order to change. Motivation stems from looking ahead and imagining either the positive results of our actions or the negative consequences of not taking action. These need to be compelling.

The positive consequences

I'm sure you can think of many benefits you could gain. For example, the positive consequences of altering your lifestyle might include a clearer mind, better concentration, greater contentment, consistent energy, relaxed muscles, a feeling of internal calmness, brighter spirits, a good appetite, better weight control, clear skin, bright eyes, glossy hair, flexible joints, regular bowels, strong teeth and good vitality.

The negative consequences

What about the negative consequences of failing to make changes? Some of these might be depression, lack of energy, constipation, inertia, weight gain, flabby muscles, stiff joints, anxiety, constant coughs and colds, loose bowels, poor sleep, poor memory, lack of appetite, constantly getting upset, irritability or general failing health.

Action Box
Remember the 'carrot' and the 'stick'

Most of us need both a positive and a negative payoff to be truly compelled to make lifestyle adjustments. If you currently have an illness that stops you from functioning well and at the same time you know you really want to enjoy your life and be healthy, you have both a carrot and a stick to motivate you. But equally you need to set realistic health goals and not become rigid or obsessed.

81 Make your goals specific and achievable

So what do you want to change about your lifestyle? If you are vague about the lifestyle improvements you want to make then you'll get vague results. Nothing will change. It's important for our outcome to be *clear, specific* and *stated in the positive* for us to achieve our goals.

If you're wondering whether you've got a positive or negative goal ask yourself if it's something you want to include or exclude. If it's something you want to include in your life it's a positive goal. If it's something you want to exclude from your life it's a negative one. It's best to know what we want to include.

You can turn a negative goal into a positive one by asking: 'If I had that what would it be like?'

Action Box
Turning negative goals into positive ones

Here are some negative outcomes changed to positive ones:

Negative outcome	**Positive outcome**
I don't want to feel so tired.	I want to be able to sustain my energy throughout the day.

I don't want to put on weight.	I want to be slim and have a well-toned body.
I don't want to feel so miserable.	I want to feel positive and optimistic.

There are a few other questions you might ask yourself just to be sure your goal is specific and achievable:

- What stops you from already having achieved your goal?
- What resources do you have that will help you to reach your goal?
- If you made these changes, would you lose anything?

It is often helpful to write down your answers to these questions.

82 Allow yourself some imperfections

Sometimes people avoid making lifestyle changes because they are frightened of failing. They go around feeling guilty for not adjusting their lifestyle as they 'should' and become stuck and unable to change as a result. It's best to remember – *you don't have to be perfect.*

It's best that we enjoy the process of change and that we each do it in our own unique way. Let's feel proud and satisfied that we are doing the best for ourselves. There is no such thing as a 'right' way of living – just some helpful golden rules that can guide us.

Action Box
Give yourself treats

Some people keep small 'treats' for themselves when they change their diet. If they're exercising they make sure they give themselves praise rather than criticizing themselves for what they can't do. Improvement sometimes comes in small, steady increments and not every part of your life has to be perfect.

83 Take teeny tiny steps

A Chinese saying states that a journey of 1,000 miles takes the first step. Any change you make doesn't have to be huge. In fact tiny adjustments often lead on to something much larger.

A friend started learning *qigong* and found it hard to get into a routine of practising. She decided to practise for just five minutes a day. She would use a timer and then stopped when five minutes were up. In time she enjoyed it so much it went up to ten minutes, fifteen minutes and then twenty minutes. At present she's practising for twenty minutes a day and has kept up the habit for a year. The results she has accrued from the regular practice are far more than if she had practised irregularly but for more hours.

Another patient thought giving up sugar might be helpful to her so she decided to stop for a month only. After that she told herself she could eat it again. After that month finished she'd changed her habits. She no longer wanted to eat the large amount of sugar she'd previously consumed. She'd changed her habit by stealth!

Action Box
Don't do too much at once

Do the smallest amount and see how that goes – and later assess how it's working. Remember it's better to do a small amount regularly than to do nothing at all or to give up because you've taken on too much.

84 Do what you find enjoyable

Why do some of us make permanent changes to our lifestyle while others have good intentions that come to nothing? The answer is complex, of course: our habits, upbringing and emotional predisposition all come into it. Overall, one of the strongest reasons for continuing our bad habits is that the alternatives we've looked at don't seem enjoyable.

The examples in the action box below are only a few of the many ways we can make our lifestyle changes enjoyable. Doing things that we don't enjoy will ultimately have a negative impact while enjoyment in itself is conducive to our overall good health.

Action Box
Choose enjoyable options

When we choose to do something new we can look for the most enjoyable option available. For example, if we decide to do more exercise we might ask ourselves: 'What exercise do I enjoy?' and 'What do I hope to get from doing it?' We may choose gentle *qi*-enhancing exercises such as *tai ji quan,* yoga or a *qigong* class or more active exercises such as dancing, a sport or learning a martial art. Others may prefer an enjoyable challenge such as walking to work or taking up cycling.

When considering our emotions we can enjoy keeping a daily journal of appreciation, creating some positive outcomes or noticing 'the importance of keeping in good humour'. We may even deliberately go to watch a funny film or to see a comedian.

If we are used to having our lunch on the run we can decide to find pleasurable ways of giving ourselves a break. We might choose to go out to a park to eat if the weather is sunny, or go out to eat at a good restaurant or to find a different space in our workplace where we can relax and enjoy our food.

85 Find healthy substitutes

Substitution can be especially helpful when we are changing our diet. For example, if you want to give up dairy products, there are now many milk substitutes in the shops. On a trip through your supermarket or whole-food shop you will probably find oat milk, quinoa milk, rice milk, soya milk or almond milk. Shopping around is important and if you are going to substitute try out alternatives to find the one you prefer.

We can also look out for different substitutes for coffee and tea. Those who decide to give up coffee may prefer not to try taking one of the coffee 'substitutes' such as Caro or Barleycup – they'll never taste like the real thing! It might be better to try out completely new tastes. We can look out for interesting herb teas – 'Lemon Zinger' or 'Revitalise tea' might take our fancy or try Rooibosch tea for a change. Alternatively we might want to change from black tea to green tea (see Secret 30 for more on the benefits of green tea).

Once you decide on the change you wish to make and start looking at the labels you may be surprised to realize what you've been eating. One patient who gave up sugar was shocked to find that frozen peas, pasta sauces and ketchup all had sugar in them. It becomes a challenge to find healthier foods and you'll become like a detective finding alternatives.

Action Box
Have fun looking for substitutes

As well as being fun, substituting foods can add variety to what we eat and drink. For a list of suggested substitutes for food and drink, see Secret 25.

---

86 Change at your own speed

Some people choose to make lifestyle changes quickly while others make small modifications bit by bit. Many people make a combination of changes – some dramatic shifts then a number of slow changes.

Making shifts too rapidly can sometimes mean that we give up and return to our previous bad habits. In this case taking a longer time to change may be our best course of action. We know that Chinese medicine teaches that balance is important in everything we do. Making changes that are extreme will tend to rebound on us. We can then easily find ourselves going back to square one. The 70% rule about exercising (see page 136) is also true in all other areas of our lifestyle.

Action Box
Deciding on what to change

Most of us will find that some alterations are easier to make than others. Often it is best to make the simplest changes first. For example, we can easily protect ourselves from the environment by wearing a scarf, changing out of wet clothes or wearing slippers. We might choose to change these things immediately. Others, like getting enough rest, changing our diet or exercising regularly, can take a longer time to become habitual.

87 See yourself changing your lifestyle

Once you have read this chapter, this exercise can be an important reference. It will help you to consolidate any lifestyle changes you choose to make. If you visualize yourself making the changes you want to make it will reinforce the lifestyle areas you wish to adopt and make them more compelling. You can do it every day. If you do it every day for two weeks you will find you naturally start to make positive changes to your lifestyle.

You can continue to do it for other lifestyle aims.

Action Box
A small exercise that can lead to big results!

This exercise will only take 5–7 minutes. Visualize yourself making a lifestyle change you desire to make:

1. Sit comfortably, close your eyes and relax.
2. Visualize or get a sense of yourself in the future making your chosen lifestyle improvement. Be slightly distanced so that you have a picture of yourself doing it rather than feeling as if you are actually doing it now. (When you have a picture of yourself it is more likely to happen in the future.)
3. Make the image of yourself bright and colourful.
4. Step into this and try it out. Do you feel comfortable with the effects of this improvement?
5. If you feel comfortable, go to step 7.
6. If you feel at all uncomfortable make adjustments. For example, if you see yourself walking to work everyday you might realize this isn't quite right for you. You may prefer to cycle or walk only on specific days.
7. Fine-tune the adjustments until you sense that you would enjoy doing this in the future.
8. Bring in any other images which enable you to know that you are enjoying what you are doing. For example, you may be with friends, you may look happy or you may be talking about what a good time you're having. Get a sense that what you see yourself doing in the future has become a normal part of your life.
9. When you are ready, open your eyes and slowly come back into the room.

88 Don't just read about it – use it!

By the time you get to the end of this book you will probably have already made some lifestyle improvements. Just knowing the importance of things such as protecting yourself from the environment, being aware of your constitution or making dietary changes can allow you to make certain adjustments quite naturally. Drawing on the action boxes will reinforce these.

Action Box
Keep supporting the changes you have made

You may want to read this book again in a few months time to support the changes you are making. The second time you read it you will probably find more adjustments fall into place quite naturally.

You may need to put a more concerted effort into making other improvements and the tips above and action boxes can help you.

If I have one wish it is that this book assists you in becoming a happier and healthier person. May you have great vitality in the future!

8 Staying Healthy and Preventing Disease

This chapter lists some lifestyle adjustments to improve or prevent many common ailments. These suggestions are not meant as a substitute for Chinese medicine treatments such as acupuncture, Chinese herbs or Chinese massage (*tuina*).

Chinese medicine treatments can be extremely effective for most of these complaints. Once treated, patients can then prevent recurrence of the problem by making appropriate lifestyle changes.

The lifestyle suggestions in this chapter are all based on what I've written in the main chapters of the book. At the end of each ailment in this chapter you will see a list of the most helpful suggestions to refer back to in the book.

These suggestions are also not an alternative to medical help when it is needed.

We'll look at the following conditions:

- anxiety and panic attacks

- asthma

- back pain

- chronic fatigue syndrome

- constipation

- colds and flu

- depression

- diabetes

- diarrhoea

- headaches and migraines

- hypertension

- indigestion

- insomnia

- joint problems

- menopausal hot flushes

- period pains

- premenstrual tension

- skin conditions.

Anxiety and panic attacks

If you are prone to anxiety or panic attacks Chinese medicine may be very helpful. You can also help to alleviate your symptoms by following the lifestyle advice below.

Lifestyle changes that may prevent or improve anxiety and panic attacks

Diet

It may come as surprise that diet has a role to play in preventing anxiety and panic attacks. This is because a lack of 'Blood'-nourishing food (see page 44) may cause us to become unsettled inside, leading to anxiety and panic attacks. This may especially affect some vegetarians. If you are a vegetarian and have anxiety or panics attacks and you have no ethical reasons for not eating animal products it may be advisable to start eating a small amount of meat, poultry or fish. This could produce tremendous benefits to your emotional health. Do not expect an immediate change as it may take a few weeks or months for the Blood to build up in the system.

Eating a nourishing diet, rich in fresh vegetables and grains, is essential for anyone who has panic attacks or anxiety, whether they are vegetarian or not. You also need to make sure that you:

- don't skip meals

- eat three meals regularly every day

- eat in a relaxed environment.

Caffeine

Excessive amounts of caffeine from drinking tea, coffee, hot chocolate and colas can also cause some people to become over-anxious. To discover whether this is having a negative effect on your health you can try cutting caffeine out for two or three weeks. At the end of this time you can assess whether there is a difference and if so you may decide to continue to exclude it from your diet.

Relaxation and rest

Sometimes if we are leading an overactive lifestyle or have a highly stressful job this can culminate in anxiety and panics. We can put aside time for relaxation before going to bed and take at least eight hours' rest in bed even if we have difficulty sleeping. It is also beneficial to ensure that we take sufficient breaks for lunch and have a rest after lunch. Our body can create better-quality Blood if we relax and rest.

Bleeding

Any bleeding can cause Blood deficiency. Women who use a coil find that they bleed profusely during their periods. This may cause the Blood to become deficient, which in turn may be an undetected cause of panics and anxiety. If this is the case, a change of contraception may be necessary. Heavy periods or bleeding during childbirth can also cause Blood deficiency and Chinese medicine recognizes that this can be a common cause of post-natal anxiety or depression.

Qigong and *tai ji quan*

Qigong and *tai ji quan* are relaxing exercises that can have a profound effect on those who feel anxious. By carrying out the gentle exercises and strengthening the *dantien* in the lower abdomen we can learn to become calmer and more settled.

Chinese medicine treatments

Acupuncture, Chinese herbs or *tuina* (Chinese massage) can all settle and calm people who have anxiety or panic attacks. If people have lost a lot of blood (for example, from childbirth or trauma) or have heavy periods, Chinese herbs or acupuncture can help to rebalance the menstrual cycle and deal with the after-effects arising from the resulting deficiency.

These lifestyle secrets may be particularly helpful if you have anxiety and panic attacks:

4   Important transformation times that can change your life

8   Strengthen your constitutional essence by breathing into the *dantien*

17   Be an 'almost' vegetarian

18   If you are vegetarian – be a well-balanced one

19   Take good-quality food

30   Drink green tea or other healthy drinks

34   Fear makes *qi* descend and worry knots the *qi*

39   Gain perspective on your emotions

42   Use talking therapy

43   Use writing therapy

49   After a miscarriage, take time to rest

55   Sleep – the best natural cure

59   Scan your body to relax

67   A simple self-exercise more effective than massage

68   Use Chinese metal balls as a simple longevity tool.

Asthma

Asthma is a disease that affects about five million people in the UK.[1] It often starts in childhood, but it can happen for the first time at any age.

Asthma affects the airways carrying air in and out of the lungs. People with asthma have sensitive airways which become irritated in some situations. The airways become narrow and sometimes produce more mucus than usual. This makes it difficult to breathe.

Chinese medicine describes asthma as *xiao chuan*. *Xiao* means wheezing and *chuan* means breathlessness. Chinese medicine teaches that there are a number of different causes for asthma including phlegm affecting the chest, weak lungs or the after-effects of a cold.

Lifestyle changes that may prevent or improve asthma

Diet

Many people with asthma have phlegm in the chest but they may be unaware of it. Cutting out phlegm and damp-forming foods, especially dairy products, which can create a lot of mucous, can often reduce asthma symptoms.

Some asthma is triggered by intolerance to certain foods or food additives. Food intolerances can occur from eating an excessive amount of one type of food over long periods or from eating food at an early age when our digestive system is not mature enough to assimilate it. If we crave one particular food this may be a sign that we are sensitive to it. We may need to give up the very food we most enjoy in order to overcome the symptoms of intolerance.

Those who think their asthma is due to a food intolerance can do the following:

1. Try removing one or more of the suspect foods from the diet completely for a few weeks.
2. Notice if the asthma recedes during this time.

186

3. If the asthma recedes, cut out the food(s) for a longer period and watch to see if the asthma abates still more.

If we eat a nourishing diet that is rich in fresh vegetables and grains, it will strengthen our overall energy and help to prevent asthma attacks.

Protection from the environment

Most asthma sufferers know that catching a cold can intensify and trigger asthma that is otherwise latent. If you are prone to asthma it is best not to leave your upper chest exposed to windy, cold or damp weather. It is also helpful to wear a scarf in windy weather, and to wear a vest and cover your hands and feet in the cold. For more about protecting yourself from the environment, read Chapter 6.

Overactivity and rest

Inhalers allow many people with asthma to lead a normal life. However, an asthma attack is also a 'signal' that there is an underlying cause that needs to be dealt with. An inhaler temporarily alleviates the symptom but does not address the cause. Sometimes the relief gained from using an inhaler allows us to do more than is within our true capacity. This can ultimately deplete our energy. Those who have asthma are advised to guard against doing too much and to take regular rests.

Emotions

Some asthma can be aggravated by stress or emotional problems. It can often be unexpressed frustration or anger but may also be grief, anxiety or other emotions. It can be useful if you try to ascertain the specific trigger. Once you know what provokes an attack examine your lifestyle and decide how best you can deal with the stress. If possible strive to avoid getting into situations that trigger the emotions. Read Chapter 4 to find other ways of dealing with emotional strains.

Qigong and other exercises

Mild exercise can often help people with asthma. If you get no exercise at all, it may be a good idea to start learning *tai ji quan* or *qigong* as this can strengthen the chest. Strong exercise is not recommended, especially if the lungs are weak, as this may put too much strain on them.

Good posture

Asthma is sometimes caused or worsened by poor posture, especially during childhood. Children can be stooping over books, sitting on wrongly adjusted seats, watching television or using computers for long periods. In these situations they may not breathe properly because they are putting undue pressure on their chests. Adjusting the posture can be beneficial in these cases. Encouraging more breaks for activity can also help to encourage proper breathing.

Pollutants

Pollutants in the air will exacerbate an asthma attack. Living in an urban area can be especially stressful on the lungs but country areas can also be polluted, especially during crop spraying. Household paint and other products containing strong chemicals can also give off noxious fumes which can trigger attacks and household cleaners can also cause problems. House dust mites are also said to be one of the most common causes of asthma attacks. People with asthma need to keep their environment free from any of these particles and pollutants.

Smoking

Anyone who has asthma is advised to stop smoking. Smoking weakens the lung energy and causes further difficulty breathing.

Chinese medicine treatments

Both acupuncture and Chinese herbs can be extremely beneficial for those suffering from asthma.

These lifestyle secrets may be particularly helpful if you have asthma:

8   Strengthen your constitutional essence by breathing into the *dantien*

11   Rely on 'economical' foods in your daily diet

12   Choose vegetables – full of rich, life-enhancing *qi*

Back pain

Chinese medicine teaches that there are many causes for back pain and acupuncture and massage (*tuina*) can be especially effective treatments. Pain from back problems can vary from a dull ache to excruciating agony. All backache can be debilitating and it is one of the commonest reasons given for absence from work in the Western world. The National Institute for Health and Clinical Excellence (NICE) issued guidelines in 2009 that acupuncture should be made available on the NHS for chronic lower-back pain.[2]

Lifestyle changes that may prevent or improve back pain

Posture

Bad posture can either cause or exacerbate a back problem. When lifting we should bend the knees rather than the back. Lifting heavy weights can also strain the back and using labour-saving devices such as shopping baskets with wheels can prevent us from developing back problems later on.

People who have back problems are advised to use chairs that support the back and try not to sit in a slumped position. Sitting incorrectly for long periods of time will exacerbate a back problem. This is especially true for people who use computers for long periods and develop back and neck problems.

The back can also become weak after prolonged periods of standing. In this case it is best to adjust our lifestyle so that we sit down more frequently. People who are in jobs which entail long periods of standing, such as nurses, teachers or shop assistants, may find it necessary to transfer to alternative, less strenuous work.

Protection from the environment

Wind, cold and damp commonly affect the lower back. For example, when we are gardening we may build up a sweat and remove clothes. This can leave the back exposed. As we cool down afterwards, the wind, cold and damp can enter the back through the open pores. Cold causes the tissues to contract creating acute pain and the wind and damp also contribute. Similar conditions affect people working on building sites, people sunning themselves on a hot day which then turns cool or getting cold after exercising and working up a sweat. Make sure you cover up the lower back to protect it from wind, cold and damp. If necessary place a hot pad or hot bottle on the back if it starts to become painful following such events.

Sleeping in a draught can also cause neck pain. Never sleep under a fan or next to an open window as wind and cold can penetrate the neck.

Rest and relaxation

Overactivity, especially when carried out under stress, can also cause backache. The stress will cause the muscles to tighten up and the strenuous activity will weaken them. Make sure that you get enough rest, especially if you are working hard physically. Sleeping in a good posture is also essential.

Emotions

The spine is the central pillar that holds us erect and our emotions are often reflected there. If the cause of a back problem is emotional then dealing with our emotions can help to clear the physical problem. For example, if we are depressed we can feel slumped inside and this can depress the spine. If we are angry we can tighten up and tense the muscles in the back. Chinese medicine associates fear with the Kidneys and the function of these organs is associated with the spine. When we are afraid we can feel 'spineless' and have a weakened back. We can also pull away from things that make us afraid and this can put a strain on our back.

Exercise

Gentle exercise such as *tai ji quan* or *qigong* can help to relax a tight back or strengthen a weak one. It is essential to do the exercises in the correct posture with the back relaxed and straight and the pelvis tilted towards the ground. Gentle stretching exercises can also be beneficial.

Strenuous exercise such as lifting weights, vigorous jogging or energetic racquet games can aggravate a back problem and anyone with a weak back should avoid these exercises.

Chinese medicine treatments

Acupuncture is an excellent treatment for many types of back pain and has been widely researched. It can deal with an acute or chronic back problem. *Tuina* (Chinese massage) can also be helpful in the treatment of back problems.

Other treatments

Although not a part of Chinese medicine, chiropractic, osteopathy and craniosacral therapy need to be mentioned here as they can also be beneficial for many back problems. The Alexander Technique can also be helpful if poor posture is the cause.

These lifestyle secrets may be particularly helpful if you have back pain:

3   Accept your limits and live within their confines

9   Strengthen your constitutional essence by sensing into the *dantien*

33   Anger makes *qi* rise

34   Fear makes *qi* descend and worry knots the *qi*

39   Gain perspective on your emotions

Chronic fatigue syndrome

Chronic fatigue syndrome or post-viral syndrome is a frequent cause of chronic illness. Symptoms can include overwhelming exhaustion that is not relieved by rest, muscle aches and weakness, concentration and memory problems, depression, bowel problems and intermittent flu-like feelings. This condition is usually caused by a combination of depleted energy and an infection or virus that remains in the body because the body is too weak to eliminate it. Chinese medicine describes this as a 'pathogenic factor' that is remaining in the body.

Lifestyle changes that may prevent or improve chronic fatigue syndrome

Prevention

The best 'treatment' for chronic fatigue syndrome is prevention. People who get this condition are often chronically overworking and weakening their body's energy. If they then catch an infection resulting in what Chinese medicine calls 'an invasion of wind, cold, heat or damp', they are not strong enough to throw this pathogen off. Proper rest during an illness and then taking time to convalesce will give the body the chance to regain its strength so that it can throw off the climatic factor/virus.

To prevent chronic fatigue syndrome it is advisable to live a lifestyle that is not overly stressful or overactive. Rest when you are tired and eat nourishing food.

Rest

Rest is essential to prevent chronic fatigue syndrome. Once someone has this condition, they feel so worn out it is impossible not to rest. Many people with this condition can't accept their change in circumstances and some find they are too restless to relax properly. Acceptance can be one of the first steps to recovery.

Diet

Eating a well-proportioned diet with a small amount of rich food and lots of grains and vegetables is strengthening to the body. Eliminating phlegm and damp-forming foods from the diet, and cutting down on heating foods if there is heat in the system, can help to clear damp or heat from the body and help recovery.

Caffeine

Many people with chronic fatigue syndrome find that cutting out caffeinated drinks such as coffee, tea, hot chocolate and colas helps to improve the condition. Caffeinated drinks make us edgy and restless, which stops us from fully resting so that we can recover.

Avoid getting infections

Protecting ourselves from extremes of wind, cold, damp and heat or changes in temperature can help us both to prevent and alleviate chronic fatigue syndrome. If a person has chronic fatigue syndrome the body may be too weak to fight an infection which gets stuck inside the body, making the condition worse.

Light exercise

Chinese exercises such as *qigong* or *tai qi quan* can be beneficial to a person who has chronic fatigue syndrome. They can often help to clear the wind, cold, damp or heat from the system. Light walking or short sessions of other light exercises can also be helpful. It is best to avoid strenuous exercise as this will weaken the *qi* and Blood.

Stress and emotions

People who are ill with chronic fatigue syndrome have often been leading a highly stressful life before getting sick. Once ill, the condition itself becomes an additional stressor and often results in impatience to get better. As chronic fatigue syndrome can linger for long periods of time it is essential for you to accept the situation you are in and to use the time to re-examine your previous way of life. If you can then make any necessary modifications to your lifestyle this will assist the healing process and enable you to remain healthy in the future.

Chinese medicine treatments

In order to recover from chronic fatigue syndrome you need to lead a healthy lifestyle. You may also benefit from the help of an acupuncturist or Chinese herbal practitioner to strengthen the body further.

These lifestyle secrets may be particularly helpful if you have chronic fatigue syndrome:

1   Conserve your constitutional essence

3   Accept your limits and live within their confines

8   Strengthen your constitutional essence by breathing into the *dantien*

10 Balance the proportions of your food

14 Don't overdose on 'rich' foods

19 Take good-quality food

25 Find tasty substitutes

30 Drink green tea or other healthy drinks

31 Be alert for food sensitivities

32 Emotions are a key to good health

38 Know the importance of humour

40 Become present to your bodily 'felt sense'

Colds and flu

If we keep ourselves healthy Chinese medicine teaches that we will have strong *wei* or defensive energy. The defensive energy lies just between the skin and muscles and protects us from the invasion of 'wind' from the environment. The defensive energy is similar to what is called the immune system in Western medicine. Colds and flu are classified either as by 'wind-cold' or 'wind-heat' in Chinese medicine (see chapter 6).

Lifestyle changes that may prevent or improve colds and flu

Protection from climatic factors

We are vulnerable to catching colds and flu when there is a change in temperature. To prevent them, we can make sure that we wear appropriate clothes when going in and out of heated buildings, when we return to a cold climate from sunny holidays or when the weather changes unseasonably.

We are also more vulnerable when we are in windy weather conditions. Chinese medicine understands that windy weather can be anything from the actual wind, to draughts, the air blowing from a fan or air conditioning. The neck area is very vulnerable to the effects of wind. When we are in these environments we especially need to cover the neck.

Stress

If we are under stress our defensive energy (and therefore the immune system) is weakened and we become vulnerable to catching colds and flu. During these stressful times in our lives we are often most neglectful of our health (see Chapter 4, page 80 for a list of common stressors in our lives). At these times we need to be particularly vigilant and make sure we eat properly and get enough rest and sleep to guard against illness.

Overwork and rest

Overwork can cause our energy to become depleted. Our defensive energy then weakens and this makes us more vulnerable to catching colds. A cold can swiftly affect everyone in our working environment, especially if the people in it are overworked and under stress.

If you become ill with a cold it is best to drop everything and rest. This will often stop the cold from developing, but if it does develop it is advisable to take time off work to convalesce. Ensure that you have fully recovered your health before returning to work and you will then be less vulnerable to more infections. It will also save your work colleagues from becoming infected and prevent an epidemic from occurring all around the building.

Clearing a cold

The Chinese medicine classification of 'wind-cold' and 'wind-heat' each needs to be dealt with in a different way.

Wind-cold
This causes symptoms such as a stuffy nose with clear white mucous, an itchy throat, sneezing, coughing, a slight headache at the base of the skull, a desire to keep warm and/or slightly achy joints.

A person who has a wind-cold needs to sweat in order to eliminate the wind from the body through the pores. A ginger tea will encourage us to sweat. To make a ginger tea:

1. Place 3–5 slices of ginger in a cup.
2. Pour boiling water in it.
3. Leave it to brew for about 5 minutes.
4. Add 1 teaspoonful of honey.

Alternatively, an old-fashioned 'hot toddy' will have the same effect. To make a hot toddy, mix together a capful of whisky with a teaspoonful of honey in boiling water. After taking these remedies it is important to keep warm while the pores are opened to let out the cold.

Wind-heat

This is often more severe than wind-cold and similar to influenza. We might feel hot and feverish as well as sweaty and thirsty and have swollen tonsils or a sore throat. We might also have a stuffy or runny nose with yellow mucous, fairly severe joint pains as well as a desire to keep warm.

A peppermint tea will help to cool the body and clear wind-heat:

1. Place 1 peppermint teabag in boiling water.
2. Add 1 teaspoonful of honey.
3. Leave for 5 minutes.

Although the best 'treatment' for a cold is prevention, once we have a cold it is important to clear it from the system. Colds that are not cleared can travel deeper into the body and weaken the lungs. Long-term use of antibiotics will also weaken our immune system and lead to weak lungs.

Chinese medicine treatments

Chinese herbal medicine can treat colds and flu and can be used both to strengthen the defensive *qi* to prevent colds and to clear colds from the body. Acupuncture can also be used in a similar way and can both treat colds and flu and help strengthen the body to prevent infections.

These lifestyle secrets may be particularly helpful if you have a tendency to get colds and flu:

1   Conserve your constitutional essence

12   Choose vegetables – full of rich, life-enhancing qi

19   Take good-quality food

35   Grief and sadness dissolve *qi*

48   Convalescence – the forgotten secret

55   Sleep – the best natural cure

73   How to prevent colds, flu and other acute problems.

Constipation

If we open our bowels less frequently than once a day or have difficulty expelling the stool then we are constipated. Some people can only open their bowels with the help of laxatives. If this is the case it is better to find natural ways to open our bowels and become less dependent on pills.

Lifestyle changes that may prevent or improve constipation

Diet

Diet is especially important in the treatment of constipation. It is best if our diet is well proportioned and full of fresh vegetables, whole grains, beans and fruit. This diet will provide fibre which is essential to normal bowel movements. Those who have a tendency to constipation need to beware of eating processed food or 'fast foods' which contain very little fibre and nourishment.

Any extremes of diet can also be the cause of constipation. We can look at our diet and notice if we are eating too much cooling or heating food or are eating too much of one taste in our diet. An excess of heating foods can dry up the stools while too much cooling food can slow them down. Excess phlegm and damp-forming food can slow down the Spleen's transforming and transporting process causing constipation (see Chapter 3 for more about diet).

Emotional stress

Unexpressed emotions or any emotional 'holding on' over long periods of time may start to reflect physically in the bowels and cause constipation. This is especially true if we are harbouring anger, resentment or frustration but can also be unexpressed grief, sadness or other emotions. Examining our lives to discover whether there are unresolved emotions may free us up mentally which may then result in the physical effect of easier bowel movements.

Exercise

A static lifestyle can cause constipation. Regular light exercise is important for anyone who is constipated as it encourages bowel movements.

Overwork

Chinese medicine theory teaches that the Spleen is responsible for all transformation and movement in the body. If we overwork we can weaken the Spleen so that it can no longer move and transform. This can cause the bowels to become sluggish. If the bowels are sluggish it is important to get enough rest and to eat in the right conditions.

Regularity

The best time to open the bowels is in the morning and it is possible to develop a regular routine each day. Some people find it difficult to open their bowels in strange environments or away from home. If the morning becomes the regular time, we will normally be opening the bowels before leaving home and this may help to overcome such problems.

Chinese medicine treatments

Chinese herbs and acupuncture can both effectively treat constipation. When necessary, however, it will also be important for patients to adjust their lifestyle habits in some of the ways suggested above.

These lifestyle secrets may be particularly helpful if you have constipation:

10 Balance the proportions of your food

11 Rely on 'economical' foods in your daily diet

12 Choose vegetables – full of rich, life-enhancing *qi*

13 Avoid too much raw and cold food

15 Know your phlegm and damp-forming food

26 Eat regular meals

27 Eat in the right conditions

32 Emotions are a key to good health

39 Gain perspective on your emotions

51 Keep your life regular

54 Walk your way to health

63 Find an exercise routine.

Depression

Chinese medicine teaches that there are many causes of depression. For example, it teaches that the Liver function is responsible for keeping our energy flowing smoothly throughout our systems. If we become frustrated, angry, resentful or hold in our emotions this may cause our energy to stop flowing freely, thus causing depression.

Feeling depressed can also be caused by our Lung or Heart energy becoming deficient, causing us to feel dull and lacking in joy and vitality. An internal heavy feeling of depression can also be caused by dampness that has prevented the energy from flowing easily (see page 159).

Lifestyle changes that may prevent or improve depression

Emotions

Depression can vary from low-grade depression to a depression that is so debilitating that it is impossible to move or function without help. It can initially be brought on by outside circumstances such as a relationship break-up, the death of a loved one, difficulties at work or financial worries.

Dealing with the emotional cause is an essential part of the healing process. When we are grief-stricken, anxious or worried our friends and family are often our greatest support and can help us by listening and allowing us to express our problems and worries.

Sometimes it is hard to say what has caused depression but, once in this state, it is hard to lift out of it. A common cause is unexpressed anger. If this emotional cause is recognized and the feelings articulated, it will often help to clear it.

Writing a daily journal or getting more perspective on our problems can also help us to deal with our feelings of depression. In some circumstances it may be best to get the help of a trained counsellor or therapist. Acupuncture or Chinese herbs can also be tremendously helpful.

Exercise and movement

Some types of depression will lift if we get moving. Any exercise including some brisk walking, swimming, playing a racquet game, *tai ji quan* or *qigong* will be helpful. If you are feeling low it is not always easy to get up and start exercising. Once you start moving, however, and the energy starts flowing again, you should feel better. A friend or partner can be a useful resource if they can persuade you to become more active.

Diet

A regular diet rich in fresh vegetables, grains and beans will help you to become healthier and to build your energy to prevent depression. Phlegm and damp-forming foods can especially block up the system and cause a person to feel heavy and lethargic. Try cutting these from your diet for a month to find out if they are exacerbating your emotional state.

Alcohol

Alcohol can be a relaxant. Many people say it frees them up and makes them feel less depressed. Long term, however, alcohol can have a depressing effect. Stagnation of the Liver energy is often a cause of depression and alcohol can increase this stagnation.

Climate

Some people are affected by damp weather and find that they become more depressed when the weather is damp and gloomy for long periods. People who live in damp houses can also become depressed. A dehumidifier in the house will help to clear the dampness from the environment. This may in turn brighten the spirits.

Chinese medicine treatments

As stated above, acupuncture, Chinese herbs and *tuina* (Chinese massage) can all be beneficial to those who are suffering with depression.

These lifestyle secrets may be particularly helpful if you tend to get depressed:

3   Accept your limits and live within their confines

11   Rely on 'economical' foods in your daily diet

14   Don't overdose on 'rich' foods

30   Drink green tea or other healthy drinks

31   Be alert for food sensitivities

32   Emotions are a key to good health

33   Anger makes *qi* rise

35   Grief and sadness dissolve *qi*

42   Use talking therapy

43   Use writing therapy

44   The importance of positive goals

45   Release your blocked feelings

Diabetes

A healthy lifestyle is an essential ingredient in both the prevention and management of diabetes. Amazingly, Chinese medical books first described the treatment of diabetes, which was called 'wasting and thirsting disease', 2,000 years ago.

There are two types of diabetes described in Western medicine: 'Type 1' diabetes and 'Type 2' diabetes. Type 1 diabetes is often diagnosed following excessive weight loss, extreme thirst, excessive appetite and frequent urination. This is often found in young people although it can affect people of any age group. It is the least common form of diabetes and affects 5–15% of those with diabetes. People with this type of diabetes will treat themselves by injecting insulin. Chinese medicine teaches that these extreme symptoms indicate that the person is overheating. Hence the name 'wasting and thirsting' disease.

Type 2 diabetes is usually slower in onset and often affects people over 40 who are overweight. Those with this type of diabetes may not show any symptoms although some people complain of vague tiredness and needing to urinate at night. It is usually detected by a urine test. The treatment of Type 2 diabetes is usually dietary or prescribed tablets. Sometimes people with Type 2 diabetes will be treated with insulin injections. More young people are now getting Type 2 diabetes as the incidence of obesity increases.[3]

Lifestyle changes that may prevent or improve diabetes

Prevention and management

The lifestyle changes required in the management of diabetes are much the same as those needed to prevent it. Chinese medicine describes the main causes of diabetes as:

- an irregular lifestyle

- poor diet

- overwork

- stress

- too much sex.

The guidelines below will help a person who has Type 1 diabetes to ensure that they remain healthy with as few side-effects as possible. It is unlikely that you will be able to manage without taking insulin, but you might have far better sugar control and possibly reduce your intake of insulin. People with Type 2 diabetes may also find that they have better control over their diabetes. Losing weight will help to consistently lower readings of your blood sugar. Some common side-effects of diabetes include kidney disease, eye problems and nerve damage. Lifestyle changes will reduce these risks.

Diet

A healthy diet is an essential part of the regime of any diabetic. Insulin-dependent diabetics need to balance their diet carefully with their insulin requirements to avoid swings in their blood sugar. The diet described in Chapter 3 is very similar to the diet now recommended to diabetics. Eating a fresh, well-proportioned diet containing grains, beans, fruit and vegetables and a smaller amount of 'richer' food can also cut down side-effects. It can also enable a non-insulin-dependent diabetic to lose weight if necessary.

A regular lifestyle

This is essential for everyone in order to have good health, but especially important if you have diabetes. Eating regularly, sleeping regular hours and getting regular exercise have all been found to increase the sugar control of a diabetic and thus improve health.

Exercise

Moderate exercise has been found to be beneficial to a diabetic. Exercise keeps the blood vessels healthier, reducing risks of circulation problems. Exercise is best done on a regular basis.

Overwork and rest

Chinese medicine suggests that people who have Type 1 diabetes have often weakened their energy by overworking for long periods. It is important for those with diabetes to take regular rest breaks during the day, including after meals, and to eat meals slowly and in restful conditions.

Sex

Chinese medicine also cites too much sex as a precipitating factor for Type 1 diabetes. Overworking can lead to the development of a large sexual appetite as a way to help the body to release stress. This can lead to weakening of the energy, and in Chinese medicine terms a depletion of the Kidney functioning.

Emotions

An emotional shock can be the precipitating factor before the onset of diabetes. Keeping healthy generally can enable a person to deal with emotional shocks and crises if they arise. If you have diabetes, remaining emotionally balanced can help you to keep your sugar well controlled.

Chinese medicine treatments

It is unlikely that a person with Type 1 diabetes will be able to come off insulin completely even with acupuncture or Chinese herbal treatment. Treatment can, however, be useful to supplement a healthy regime and help a person with diabetes to maintain their health. People with Type 2 diabetes who take tablets may be able to reduce them with the help of these treatments.

These lifestyle secrets may be particularly helpful if you have diabetes:

3   Accept your limits and live within their confines

6   Looking after the affairs of the bedroom

9   Strengthen your constitutional essence by sensing into the *dantien*

10   Balance the proportions of your food

11   Rely on 'economical' foods in your daily diet

12   Choose vegetables – full of rich, life-enhancing *qi*

Diarrhoea

It is normal to pass a well-formed stool every day. If the stools are semi-formed or watery and we open our bowels more than once or twice a day then we have diarrhoea. If we have chronic diarrhoea we will not get enough nourishment from our food. Long term this weakens our overall energy

Lifestyle changes that may prevent or improve diarrhoea

Diet

One of the most common causes of loose bowels is too much cold food in our diet. Chinese medicine teaches that the Spleen likes 'warmth'. If we eat too much cold food the Spleen can't work efficiently and our food is not digested well. Cold food includes any food that is eaten straight from the fridge such as iced drinks, ice cream or yoghurts. It is better to take food or drink at room temperature. Cold food also includes fruits that are cold in nature and too many raw vegetables which can also be hard to digest.

Excessive amounts of sweet food can also weaken the Spleen and this can exacerbate loose bowels.

If you are prone to diarrhoea you can strengthen your digestive system by eating regularly and taking a healthy diet with the correct proportions of grains and vegetables and only small quantities of rich foods. Cut down on phlegm and damp-forming foods such as dairy produce. It is best to avoid fast food or other poor-quality food as these weaken the digestion.

Eating too much greasy and heating food such as strong curries or excessive fatty meat such as lamb or beef sometimes causes acute, extremely foul-smelling diarrhoea. Eating contaminated food can also cause acute diarrhoea – we should take care to observe proper food hygiene.

Climate

Loose bowels can be caused by excessive cold, heat or dampness. It is often fashionable during hot weather to leave the stomach and abdomen uncovered by wearing a bikini or a short blouse. If this area is unprotected and the weather becomes cold then the cold can penetrate the stomach and abdomen causing acute and painful diarrhoea. Walking around with bare feet means the cold can travel up the legs to the intestines causing acute diarrhoea. Sitting on damp grass can allow dampness to penetrate the lower abdomen directly, causing loose bowels.

Emotions

Short episodes of worry or slight stress can result in loose bowels that clear once the stress has gone. If we are under constant stress, however, in our home or work situation this can result in chronic diarrhoea that can be very depleting. By dealing with the cause of the stress our diarrhoea can be eliminated.

Overwork or overactivity

Constantly working for long hours without rest, or over-exercising can both deplete our Spleen energy and cause loose bowels. If you have chronic loose bowels you can benefit from eating in restful conditions and taking a short nap after eating. This will help the Spleen to transform your food so that it can nourish you.

Chinese medicine treatments

Acupuncture, Chinese herbs or *tuina* (Chinese massage) can all be helpful in the treatment of diarrhoea. Treatment can smooth and strengthen the energy and allow the digestion to normalize. The lifestyle suggestions above can help to ensure the normal bowel action is maintained.

These lifestyle secrets may be particularly helpful if you tend to have diarrhoea:

10   Balance the proportions of your food

13   Avoid too much raw and cold food

15   Know your phlegm and damp-forming food

19   Take good-quality food

22   Know the temperature of your food

34   Fear makes *qi* descend and worry knots the *qi*

39   Gain perspective on your emotions

47   Balance *yin* and *yang* in your work and rest

55   Sleep – the best natural cure

71   Cold can cause of infertility and other lower-body symptoms

75   Protect yourself from the effects of damp.

Headaches and migraines

There are many types of headaches. They can occur on different parts of the head, have varying types of pain and be experienced at a range of intensities. Chinese medicine teaches a simple way of classifying headaches by noticing whether they are 'full' or 'empty' in their nature.

A 'full' headache is sometimes classed as a migraine and is often described as throbbing, boring, stabbing, pulling, distending or heavy. These pains are often severe and the headache can be very debilitating. The positions of these headaches are varied and can be situated on the temples, at the sides or top of the head or behind the eyes.

A 'deficient' headache is often described as a weak, dull or empty headache. The pain is less intense and is often an empty feeling inside the head, or is at the back of the neck, on the forehead or at the top of the head.

Chinese medicine teaches that headaches have many different causes and differentiates at least 12 types of headaches.

Lifestyle changes that may prevent or improve headaches

The two most common triggers for headaches are diet or stress, although general lifestyle can also be important.

Diet

Diet can play an important part in helping to relieve headaches. Some headaches are exacerbated by one food. We can use this simple method to find out if a food is causing headaches or is making them worse:

1. Choose one or two foods that are frequently taken in the diet and stop eating them for a period of four to six weeks.
2. Notice if the frequency of the headaches reduces during this time.
3. If your headaches have not reduced reintroduce the foods and choose one or two new foods to stop eating for a further four to six weeks.
4. Continue isolating different foods until you have found the major triggers.

The most common triggers for headaches cited by Western doctors are cheese, chocolate and oranges and it is indeed a good idea to begin by cutting these foods from your diet. Coffee and tea can also set off headaches. You might benefit from cutting alcohol from your diet. Alcohol is very 'hot' in nature and it can cause a headache from too much 'heat' going to the head. Heating foods such as curries and red meats can also cause headaches.

A diet high in rich and greasy food or phlegm and damp-forming food can be the cause a certain kind of headache and result in a heavy feeling across the forehead. A dull headache on the forehead or at the top of the head can be caused by Blood deficiency. For those who are vegetarian, a diet that contains animal protein may help stop the headaches. Those who don't wish to eat meat need to be especially careful to eat a diet rich in Blood-nourishing food.

A poor-quality diet or not eating enough food can also be the cause of headaches, so you are advised to make sure you eat well and at regular intervals.

Emotions and stress

A headache can be a 'message' that we are under stress. Pent-up frustration and anger, excessive worrying, anxiety or fear can all be the cause of headaches. If our emotions are unexpressed over a period of time they can build up until they explode into a headache. Women may get headaches before a period when they are most tense. Some people find that they get headaches after a period of stress is over, when they are resting. This often occurs at the weekend.

If you are prone to headaches caused by stress you need to isolate the cause of the tension. Once you discover which situations can provoke a headache you can avoid the trigger as much as possible and also deal with the underlying cause (see Chapter 4 for dealing with our emotions).

Too much mental work

People with jobs that involve thinking or concentrating for long periods of time can be prone to headaches. This includes those who are studying, working with computers, or who do large amounts of reading. Eye or neck strain caused by the mental work can also cause a headache. If you do this kind of mental work try to take five-minute rest breaks every hour. Gently rotating the neck in clockwise and anti-clockwise circles will help to reduce neck strain and also relaxes the eyes.

Overwork or too much exercise

Overworking can weaken your energy and cause headaches. If you notice that your headaches come on or intensify when you work harder, then you might need to cut down on what you are doing.

Chinese medicine treatments

Acupuncture has been well researched as an effective treatment of headaches. The outcome has been as high as 92% responding positively to treatment in one research trial.[4] *Tuina* (Chinese massage) and Chinese herbs can also be helpful.

These lifestyle secrets may be particularly helpful if you tend to get headaches:

8   Strengthen your constitutional essence by breathing into the *dantien*

15   Know your phlegm and damp-forming food

17   Be an 'almost' vegetarian

23   Not *too* hot or cold – keep it balanced

31   Be alert for food sensitivities

33   Anger makes *qi* rise

37   Take pleasure from the world

38   Know the importance of humour

45   Release your blocked feelings

47   Balance *yin* and *yang* in your work and rest

56   Sleep in a healthy posture.

Hypertension

The Chinese medicine classics did not describe the treatment of hypertension. High blood pressure is measured using a sphygmomanometer. A sphygmomanometer was first invented in the late 19th century long after many of these texts were written. Headaches, dizziness, irritability or a slight ringing in the ears are all signals of high blood pressure, however, and their treatment has been described.

Often people don't have any obvious signs and symptoms and only discover that their blood pressure is high when it is measured by a doctor or Chinese medicine practitioner. Long-term chronic high blood pressure can cause a stroke or a heart attack.

Lifestyle changes that may prevent or improve hypertension

Common lifestyle causes of hypertension are a combination of stress, diet and lack of rest and relaxation. If people learn to deal with these areas they can often successfully lower their blood pressure.

211

Warning: People on blood-pressure medication should only cut it down under the guidance of their doctor.

Emotional stress

Stress that causes frustration, resentment or explosive anger can be a major reason for hypertension by causing the system to become overactive. Finding ways to deal with the angry feelings can be essential in reducing blood pressure.

Diet

Too much rich, fatty food in the diet is a common cause of high blood pressure. Cutting out phlegm and damp-forming food, especially dairy produce such as milk, butter and cheese, as well as fatty meat products and any other rich food such as mayonnaise, ice cream and rich cakes and biscuits can help to lower the blood pressure.

Salt

It is advisable to cut down on your salt intake. Salt regulates the water balance in the body but in large quantities it will stress the heart and kidneys and intensify high blood pressure.

Alcohol

Chinese medicine teaches that alcohol is very heating and over-consumption can create too much heat in the body. This in turn can raise the blood pressure. For those who are drinking on a daily basis, cutting down or cutting out alcohol can help to lower the blood pressure.

Relaxation

Anything that relaxes you will help to bring down your blood pressure. This could include meditation, relaxation exercises or listening to relaxing music. Some people find that buying a relaxation tape enables them to unwind and rest and this in turn helps to lower the blood pressure. Gentle exercises such as *qigong* and *tai ji quan* can also be beneficial.

Overwork

Overworking can put the body under such strain that it raises blood pressure. In this case the hypertension is a signal to reassess the way that you are working and to relax more.

Chinese medicine treatments

Acupuncture and Chinese herbs can be very beneficial in the treatment of high blood pressure. The Chinese medicine practitioner will monitor the effects of the treatment and, if necessary, will work with the general practitioner when treating this condition.

These lifestyle secrets may be particularly helpful if you have hypertension:

8   Strengthen your constitutional essence by breathing into the *dantien*

14 Don't overdose on 'rich' foods

24 Blend the tastes of your food

32 Emotions are a key to good health

33 Anger makes *qi* rise

37 Take pleasure from the world

38 Know the importance of humour

39 Gain perspective on your emotions

50 The positive effects of fulfilling work

58 Make time for rest and relaxation

59 Scan your body to relax

62 Know the 70% principle for all activity.

Indigestion

Symptoms of indigestion include discomfort and/or pain in the stomach, feeling full, sour regurgitation or belching. Chinese medicine teaches that this is due to internal stagnation causing the normal digestive process temporarily to stop.

Lifestyle changes that may prevent or improve indigestion

The main causes of indigestion are an overly rich diet, overeating, eating in a hurry, unexpressed anger or worry.

Diet

Anyone who frequently gets indigestion is advised to examine their diet. If the diet contains too high a percentage of rich food then reducing this to 10–15% can help to alleviate the problem. Overeating can also cause indigestion, in which case the diet needs to be modified.

If you get indigestion, also strive to eat in situations which are as stress-free and as calm as possible and to continue to relax for a little while after eating in order to aid the digestive process.

Emotions

If you are griped by anxiety, fear, worry or dread it can affect the solar plexus and stomach. This may cause the digestive process to come to a temporary standstill.

Unexpressed anger and resentment can also cause our digestion to slow down or come to a standstill. Once the problem has been resolved the digestion will start moving again. Long-term resentment or anger that has not been resolved can cause chronic indigestion. These feelings may be resolved when you explore their origins and learn to let go of them.

Some people with digestive problems find themselves in situations that they find hard to sort out and 'digest'. In this case they may need to observe the situation closely in order to find the best way to deal with it and 'digest' it thoroughly.

Chinese medicine treatments

Acupuncture, Chinese herbs and *tuina* (Chinese massage) can all be used to treat indigestion and many other digestive problems. Chinese herbs travel directly to the gut. In some cases this may be beneficial and treatment may help us to digest food better. In other cases acupuncture or *tuina* may be preferable treatment as they by-pass the digestion and work directly on our energy.

These lifestyle secrets may be particularly helpful if you are prone to indigestion:

10 Balance the proportions of your food

11 Rely on 'economical' foods in your daily diet

12 Choose vegetables – full of rich, life-enhancing *qi*

13 Avoid too much raw and cold food

14 Don't overdose on 'rich' foods

15 Know your phlegm and damp forming food

26 Eat regular meals

27 Eat in the right conditions

31 Be alert for food sensitivities

34 Fear makes *qi* descend and worry knots the *qi*

40 Become present to your bodily 'felt sense'

47 Balance *yin* and *yang* in your work and rest

51 Keep your life regular

58 Make time for rest and relaxation

71 Cold can cause of infertility and other lower-body symptoms.

Insomnia

Insomnia is the inability to get off to sleep or waking in the night having initially fallen asleep.

Lifestyle changes that may prevent or improve insomnia

Emotions

Many of us have the occasional time when we go to bed worried, anxious or angry and find we can't sleep. If this happens frequently it may be time to examine your lifestyle and deal with the cause of our emotional upsets. See anxiety and worry earlier in this chapter but, for more on dealing with our emotions generally, see Chapter 4.

Overwork and rest

Many people who overwork, especially in a stressful environment, find that when they go to bed they can't sleep. Before going to bed make sure that you have wound down so that you are relaxed. Go for a quiet walk, have a relaxing bath, listen to a relaxation tape, meditate or do any other restful activity. Make sure you don't over-stimulate yourself before bed by carrying out activities such as strenuous exercise, watching a scary film, using your computer or reading over-stimulating books.

Diet

Eating irregularly or late at night can cause insomnia by putting a strain on the stomach and intestines which are having to digest food when they should be resting. Overeating on a regular basis can also mean you find it difficult to sleep, as can eating too much rich food such as puddings and sweets.

Too much hot food such as curries, red meats or alcohol can overheat a person and cause insomnia.

For vegetarians, adding some meat or protein to the diet can help to nourish the Blood and settle you.

Caffeine

Drinking large amounts of coffee, tea and colas can mean that the caffeine prevents sleep. Cutting down or cutting out these drinks and replacing them with herb teas, coffee substitutes or hot water can also help to induce sleep.

Sleeping times

People who have insomnia are advised to go to bed at a regular time every night. Our body then gets into the habit of preparing to sleep at this time. One old wives' tale tells us that the hours before midnight are twice as beneficial to us as the hours after midnight. Rest and sleep are vital for our wellbeing and getting to bed well before midnight will ensure that we get nourishing sleep.

Posture and direction

Sleeping on our side will take the pressure off our internal organs. This can prevent illness later in life. Sleeping with the head pointing towards the north helps some people to sleep more deeply as they are then aligned to the earth's magnetic field.

Blood loss

Blood loss from heavy periods (sometimes as a result of using a coil) or following an accident or birth can cause Blood deficiency. This can cause restlessness, creating insomnia. Eating a healthy diet full of Blood-nourishing foods will help to remedy this. Chinese medicine especially suggests a nourishing chicken soup after giving birth. If the blood loss is due to using the coil then it may be important to change the type of contraception.

Chinese medicine treatments

Acupuncture and Chinese herbs can both be effective treatment for insomnia. It is important for the patient to follow any of the lifestyle advice above or on page 123 to ensure that the sleep pattern is stabilized.

These lifestyle secrets may be particularly helpful if you are prone to insomnia:

17 Be an 'almost' vegetarian

18 If you are vegetarian – be a well-balanced one

23 Not *too* hot or cold – keep it balanced

26 Eat regular meals

27 Eat in the right conditions

30 Drink green tea or other healthy drinks

32 Emotions are a key to good health

33 Anger makes *qi* rise

Joint problems

The heading 'joint pains' covers a large number of conditions that include rheumatoid arthritis, osteoarthritis, bursitis, fibrositis, etc. This also covers an injury to a joint or a joint that is 'worn out'. Sometimes only one joint at a time is affected. Inflamed joints such as those found in rheumatoid arthritis are more severe and several joints will be affected.

Chinese medicine views joint pain in a different way from Western medicine. Joint pains can be caused by either a 'full' condition that needs to be cleared from the system or a 'deficient' condition that needs to be strengthened.

'Full' joint pains

Wind in the joints is characterized by pain in the muscles and joints which moves from place to place. *Cold* in the joints causes severe pain that creates limitation of movement. *Dampness* in the joints is characterized by stiffness and swelling along with a feeling of heaviness in the joint or limb. *Heat* in the joints causes them to become red, swollen, hot and painful.

When the joints have been affected for a long period of time the fluids dry up causing nodules to form. Chinese medicine calls these '*phlegm*' *nodules*.

'Deficient' joint pains

If our energy is deficient this can cause the joints to be achy rather than painful. The limbs may also feel weak.

Lifestyle changes that may prevent or improve joint conditions

Protection from the environment

Wind, cold or damp can enter the body from the outside. If you already have joint problems caused by wind, damp, cold, etc., you are often more susceptible to the external climate.

Damp in the joints will often mean you are vulnerable to damp or humid weather. People with this condition often know when the weather is turning damp because of the achy feeling they experience. In the same way, wind or cold can also exacerbate joint pains. Extremely hot weather can also worsen red, hot, swollen joints.

We can protect ourselves from these climatic conditions as much as possible by wearing appropriate clothing and living in a healthy environment.

Diet

The right diet can have a beneficial effect on the joints. A healthy diet which is rich in fresh vegetables and fruit as well as grains and beans, with only a small amount of fat, can have a strengthening effect so that you feel less weakened by your condition.

Try to notice if your joints seem to be more damp, hot or cold. Then try cutting out excessively hot or cold foods or any rich or phlegm and damp-forming foods accordingly. Drinking excessive amounts of orange juice can also exacerbate some joint conditions.

Trauma

An injury to a joint may be the precursor to a later joint problem. An injured joint should be rested to make sure it heals properly before it is used again. An injury that doesn't heal completely is vulnerable to the climatic factors of wind, cold and damp. These can easily enter an injured joint causing arthritis later on in life.

Emotions

An emotional crisis or shock can trigger arthritis. The trigger can be the death of a loved one, redundancy, divorce or financial problems or any other life crisis.

This kind of shock may cause a large number of joints to become inflamed. Of course we can't tell when a crisis is coming our way and the best way to guard against the worst effects of this kind of situation is to keep as healthy as possible. We can do this by eating, sleeping and resting regularly and by keeping a positive attitude to life as much as possible.

Exercise

Regular, gentle exercise such as *tai ji quan* or *qigong* are often beneficial to our joints and can help our mobility. It will also strengthen our underlying energy which can be weakened by the arthritic condition. These exercises are gentle and don't strain the joints. Vigorous exercise such as running or playing racquet games can strain the joints and will not be of benefit to people who have arthritic conditions or joint problems.

Swimming can often be helpful to someone with joint pains as the water protects the joints while they are exercised. If you have damp or cold in the joints, however, you should guard against getting cold when leaving the pool or not getting dry properly as this can sometimes cause further 'invasions' of cold and damp.

Rest

Some joint problems are caused by overuse of one particular area. For example if you are constantly carrying heavy loads your hips may be affected. A footballer may get bad knees. People working on computers may get problems with their neck, hands and wrists – a symptom commonly known as Repetitive Strain Injury or RSI. If one area is affected by overuse then it is advisable to rest this area as much as possible so that it can heal. This may prevent further problems arising in the future. A change of job may even be necessary if the problem does not subside.

Chinese medicine treatments

So effective is acupuncture and *tuina* (Chinese massage) in the treatment of joint problems that they are often the first treatments used by people in China. Chinese herbs can also be helpful.

These lifestyle secrets may be particularly helpful if you have joint pains:

9   Strengthen your constitutional essence by sensing into the *dantien*

Menopausal hot flushes

The most common cause of menopausal hot flushes is what Chinese medicine calls 'depletion of the *yin* energy'. *Yin* is cooling, moistening and calming. *Yang* on the other hand is heating, drying and moving (see page 110). As we grow older we need to rest appropriately. Many of us continue to overwork when we need to rest and this uses up the *yin* energy. We are left with too little of this cooling energy and too much hot energy, causing hot flushes.

It may be useful for women who have hot flushes to keep a journal of situations that have occurred just prior to the hot flush. This will then enable them to understand what has triggered the flush. Triggers are often one or more of the things listed below.

Lifestyle changes that may prevent or improve menopausal hot flushes

Overwork and rest

It is now normal for many people to overwork in ways they never did before. Overwork can wear out our *yin* energy. Hot flushes when they first appear can be a signal that you need to rest. If you take notice of this signal and really reduce your activity the flushes will often reduce in their intensity. It is interesting to note that in the past hot flushes were not as common in China as in the West. This may have changed as Chinese people's lifestyles become more Westernized. Resting may involve cutting down on work, getting enough sleep or finding ways to relax such as meditation or relaxation exercises.

Diet

If you are getting hot flushes it is best to avoid eating too many heating foods. These include red meats such as beef and lamb, curries, alcohol and coffee.

Stress and emotions

Repressed emotions such as anger and frustration can result in a build-up of heat in the body. If you can discharge these emotions you may feel able to 'cool off' and the flushes may then reduce in frequency.

Climate

A hot climate, although not usually the cause of hot flushes, can exacerbate them so that they intensify. If you have hot flushes try to avoid situations where you will be hot for long periods such as working in hot kitchens, going away to very hot climates or having saunas. If the heat is unavoidable then it is best to protect yourself as much as possible by wearing cotton clothes that allow you to sweat and to wear a hat to protect your head from the sun.

Chinese medicine treatments

Both acupuncture and Chinese herbs can nourish a person's *yin* energy and help to reduce menopausal hot flushes.

These lifestyle secrets may be particularly helpful if you have menopausal hot flushes:

4   Important transformation times that can change your life

11   Rely on 'economical' foods in your daily diet

Period pains

Chinese medicine describes many different types of period pains. The main ones are:

Pains from cold that are sharp and 'biting' in their nature. These are often better with the application of heat.

Pains that create a distended (bloated) feeling. These are often caused by stagnation in the lower abdomen. Rubbing the lower abdomen will encourage the *qi* to move and will help to alleviate the pain.

Pains that are extremely intense and do not easily respond to any massage or heat and may be accompanied by blood clots. Chinese medicine teaches that these may be due to 'stuck Blood' in the lower abdomen.

Lifestyle changes that may prevent or improve period pains

Protection from the environment

Protect yourself against cold or damp conditions by not sitting on stone steps or metal seats which may cause cold and damp to enter the lower abdomen. Also avoid leaving the abdomen uncovered and always wear shoes or slippers when walking on cold floors. Young girls playing school sports outside in cold fields wearing only shorts can suffer from cold entering the lower abdomen causing period pains due to cold.

If period pains are caused by cold in the lower abdomen then the application of heat will help temporarily. A hot water bottle or hot pad can be placed over the site of the pain.

Sex

It is best to avoid sex during a period as the uterus is at its most fragile and is more susceptible to the climate, especially to the cold. The cold can then cause period pains.

Massage

Lightly rubbing the abdomen will help some period pains. This moves the energy and in turn alleviates the pain.

Diet

If the period pains are due to cold in the lower abdomen, then it is best to avoid cold food. This includes iced drinks or food taken straight from the fridge, salad and raw food, and cold fruits. Add more warming foods to the diet by taking a moderate amount of meat and eating other hot food such as a small amount of ginger added to hot water or porridge.

Stress

Living or working in a situation which is stressful can exacerbate period pains especially those caused by stagnation. Often factors such as cold, stress and diet can all combine to intensify the condition. If you recognize that emotions play a large part in your discomfort, dealing with the cause of the stress may be the first step to alleviating the pain (see Chapter 4 for more on the emotions).

Chinese medicine treatments

Period pains due to 'stuck Blood' are extreme pains that may not respond to a change in lifestyle. In this case it is best to seek acupuncture or Chinese herbal medicine. Other types of period pains will also respond to these treatments and the lifestyle changes suggested will then keep the pains from recurring.

These lifestyle secrets may be particularly helpful if you have period pains:

9   Strengthen your constitutional essence by sensing into the *dantien*

13   Avoid too much raw and cold food

22   Know the temperature of your food

32   Emotions are a key to good health

53   Exercise while you work

54   Walk your way to health

58   Make time for rest and relaxation

59   Scan your body to relax

67   A simple self-exercise more effective than massage

70   Your pain might be caused by cold!

Premenstrual tension

The main cause of premenstrual tension is stagnation of the Liver energy. As stated earlier in the chapter, Chinese medicine teaches that the Liver is responsible for the smooth and even movement of energy throughout the body. If the Liver is not smoothing the energy it moves unevenly causing us to feel erratic, angry and irritable as well as having the other symptoms described below.

The main symptoms of this condition are fluctuating moods, depression or anger before the period, tender or swollen breasts and a swollen abdomen. Women usually begin to feel premenstrual three to four days before their period begins. Sometimes premenstrual tension can start as early as two weeks before a period. In this case it is very debilitating.

Lifestyle changes that may prevent or improve premenstrual tension

Stress and emotions

If you have premenstrual syndrome you may notice that additional difficulties during the preceding month can worsen the premenstrual symptoms while, if the month tends to run smoothly, the premenstrual tension is better. Whatever is happening either exacerbates or alleviates the quality of the premenstrual tension. Dealing with any unresolved issues in our lives can be essential to lessening the effects of this condition.

Rest

Taking a rest for half an hour every day can help you to relax. This allows the Liver energy to move and can help to clear premenstrual conditions.

Tea and coffee

Caffeinated drinks can cause us to become tense and agitated, so cutting out caffeinated drinks can help to lessen the effects of premenstrual syndrome.

Exercise

Light exercise gets the energy moving and can have a profound effect on clearing premenstrual tension. Gentle exercises such as *qigong* or *tai ji quan* can be helpful as well as brisk walking, swimming, dancing and other sports.

Chinese medicine treatments

Many women coming for treatment with acupuncture and Chinese herbs find their premenstrual tension improves. Sometimes the main complaint has been a different condition and, as the patient's overall energy becomes stronger, the premenstrual problems lessen as well.

These lifestyle secrets may be particularly helpful if you are prone to premenstrual tension:

3   Accept your limits and live within their confines

30 Drink green tea or other healthy drinks

32 Emotions are a key to good health

33 Anger makes *qi* rise

40 Become present to your bodily 'felt sense'

45 Release your blocked feelings

Skin conditions

There are many different skin conditions – eczema, psoriasis, herpes zoster, dermatitis and urticaria, to name a few. It is not within the capacity of this book to go into diagnostic details of every one of these conditions nor is it necessary. A general Chinese medicine diagnosis can be made by observing the skin.

Most skin conditions are a combination of an underlying weakness in our energy and/or Blood and external causes such as wind, cold, damp or heat affecting the skin. For example, wind will cause rashes that move around and come and go. These can be itchy and bleed, then scabs will form and they will heal up and go away again. Damp causes discharges, blisters and suppuration from the skin; there can also be puffy skin and swelling. Heat creates red, raised, painful skin conditions with a clear margin between the good skin and the diseased skin. Cold creates pale-coloured skin conditions that are better with heat.

There may also be an underlying deficiency that causes many skin conditions. In this case the main symptoms may be dry and flaky skin. Chinese medicine teaches that the Lung and skin are connected. If the Lung energy is weak this may cause many skin conditions.

Lifestyle changes that may prevent or improve skin conditions

Diet and emotions are the two most common causes of skin conditions.

Diet

A change in diet can often make a great difference to skin problems. We can adjust our diet according to what kind of skin condition is present and we can also identify any individual foods that may trigger the skin problem.

If you have a skin problem you are advised to consider the proportions of foods that you are taking in your diet. A lot of extremely rich food, including spicy food, overly sweet food or fatty food, means your diet is unbalanced. It is also advisable to restore the balance by eating plenty of freshly cooked vegetables.

If a skin problem is due to heat then it is best to avoid heating foods in the diet. These include lamb and other red meats, alcohol and hot curries that will heat the skin further. Seafoods such as mussels, lobsters, shrimps and prawns are warm-temperature foods and can trigger hot skin conditions. If you have a hot skin condition, add slightly cooling foods to the diet but not in excess.

If a skin problem is due to dampness then it is sensible to cut out or cut down on phlegm and damp-forming foods, especially dairy produce and fatty foods.

Chinese medicine teaches that Blood moistens the skin. Dry skin, which is often found in eczema and psoriasis, can be due to a deficiency of Blood. In this case a healthy diet rich in Blood-nourishing food can help to lessen the Blood deficiency and will in time benefit the skin.

A skin condition can be triggered by one or two foods taken in the diet. To ascertain which food is causing the problem cut out the suspected foods for a few weeks and notice if the skin condition starts to abate.

Emotions

Unresolved emotional problems can make us feel uncomfortable. If this discomfort is not resolved it may begin to reflect in our skin. Strong emotions, especially anger, can cause heat in the body and create red, raised, painful skin conditions. Anxiety and worry can result from Blood deficiency and create dry or flaky skin. As stated earlier Chinese medicine recognizes that the skin is the manifestation of the Lungs. Grief is the emotion connected to the Lungs and unexpressed grief can also result in skin problems.

Climate

Externally hot situations, including hot baths, can exacerbate hot skin conditions and cold skin problems can feel worse in cold weather. The skin protects us from the outside elements and if the Lung's defensive (*wei*) energy is weak the climatic causes can easily penetrate beneath the surface of the skin contributing to skin conditions.

Chinese medicine treatments

Skin conditions can be treated by any Chinese medicine treatments but Chinese herbs are certainly the most tried and tested remedy and often have a remarkable effect. It is often best to combine lifestyle adjustments with Chinese herbal treatments for the care of many skin conditions, especially severe cases.

These lifestyle secrets may be particularly helpful if you are prone to skin conditions:

10 Balance the proportions of your food

18 If you are vegetarian – be a well-balanced one

19 Take good-quality food

22 Know the temperature of your food

23 Not *too* hot or cold – keep it balanced

24 Blend the tastes of your food

31 Be alert for food sensitivities

32 Emotions are a key to good health

72 A well-kept secret – the effects of 'wind'

75 Protect yourself from the effects of damp

76 Dryness – of course it dries you up!

77 Know how to beat the heat.

This chapter has provided lifestyle suggestions for many common conditions. Even if your complaint is not mentioned in this chapter, following the guiding principles written in the main text of the book will enable you to discover how to live more healthily. This may help you to deal with your ailment and prevent other illnesses.

Notes

Chapter 1: You Can Be Really Well

1 K. T. Khaw et al., 'The Combined Impact of Health Behaviours and Mortality in Men and Women', *Public Library of Science Medicine Journal*, January 2008.
2 The 1991 Census, *Limiting Long-term Illness for Great Britain*, HMSO, 1993, Table 3.
3 Unfortunately with the increasing modernization of China many of these secrets of a healthy lifestyle are now being lost.

Chapter 2: The Secret of Respecting Our Constitution

1 Please note that these signs and symptoms can have other causes. For example, there are numerous causes cited in Chinese medicine of infertility and impotence and these symptoms can often respond to Chinese medicine treatments.
2 Many people have noticed that puberty is getting earlier – we do not know the exact reason for this and it is a slightly worrying trend. Some theories put forward are hormones in water, and animals fed on antibiotics and other drugs, including hormones.
3 B. K. L. Pillsbury, 'Doing the Month', *Health and Disease*, Open University Press, 1980, pp. 19–24.
4 G. Maciocia, *The Foundations of Chinese Medicine*, Churchill Livingstone, 2006, pp 274–5. Taken from the *Classic of a Simple Girl* (Sui Dynasty, 581–618 CE).
5 For more on breathing, see Bruce K. Frantzis, *Relaxing into your Being*.
6 For more on posture and standing meditation, see Bruce K. Frantzis, *Opening the Energy Gates of Your Body*.
7 *Gua* means the scrape. *Sha* is redness or red spots arising from the scraping.
8 My thanks to Xiao Y. Zhang who originally taught me this technique.

Chapter 3: Dietary Secrets

1 Note that modernization of China means that this 'typical' Chinese diet may be eaten less by younger Chinese people.

2 A. Bruce, 'Nutrition and Human Health', *Environment Lifestyle and Health*, a report from the European Workshop on the Environment Lifestyle and Health, Stromsted. Swedish Council for Planning and Co-ordinating Research, 1991.

3 B. Steen, 'Social Environment and Health in the Elderly', *Environment Lifestyle and Health*, a report from the European Workshop on the Environment Lifestyle and Health, Stromsted. Swedish Council for Planning and Co-ordinating Research, 1991.

4 Please note that this is approximate. Some people suggest a slightly higher proportion of vegetables and others a higher proportion of grains.

5 D. H. Buss, 'How Healthy is the British Diet?', *Journal of the Institute of Health Education*, 33(1), 1995.

6 The Japanese diet contains large amounts of rice, soya products, vegetables and fruit as well as some seaweed. A limited amount of red meat is eaten and comparatively more fish, poultry and seafood are taken. The diet also contains few dairy foods, eggs and sugar.

7 The Mediterranean diet was typical of that eaten in Crete and much of the rest of Greece and southern Italy in the early 1960s. It contained an abundance of fruit, vegetables, breads and other cereals, potatoes, beans, nuts and seeds. Olive oil was the principal source of fat. Dairy products were kept low. Fish and poultry were eaten in low to moderate amounts and red meat in low quantities too. Zero to four eggs were taken per week. Wine was also consumed in low to moderate amounts.

8 This is not necessarily the case now since proportions in the diet have changed.

9 W. C. Willett et al., 'The Mediterranean Diet Pyramid: A Cultural Model for Healthy Eating', *American Journal of Clinical Nutrition*, 61, 1995.

10 Ibid.

11 *The Balance of Good Health*, Department of Health and the Ministry of Agriculture Fisheries and Food, 1994. They now suggest a diet using these quantities of foods.

12 Xu Xiangcai, *Traditional Chinese Health Secrets*, YMAA Publication Centre, 2001, p. 10.

13 Please note that the organs and some other words such as blood have slightly different meanings if used in a Chinese medicine context rather than a Western medicine one. With this in mind I have capitalized all Organs used in a Chinese medicine context and used lower case if I am using them in a Western medicine context.

14 Tofu and miso are becoming increasingly popular healthy foods in the West. The fermenting process by which they are made helps to make them easy to digest.

15 S. Fallon and M. G. Enig, 'Tragedy and Hype: The Third International Soy Symposium', *Nexus Magazine*, 7(3), April–May, 2000.

16 T. F. H. Schmidt and R. H. Noack, 'Homeostasis', *Lifestyle Changes – A Public Health Perspective*, November 1994.

17 'Fruit and Vegetable Intakes and Prostate Cancer Risk', *Journal of National Cancer Institute*, 92(1), 5 January 2000, pp. 61–8.

18 G. Young, *The Wisdom of the Chinese Kitchen*, Simon and Schuster, 1999, pp. 33–6.

19 Bob Flaws, *Arisal of the Clear*, Blue Poppy Press, 1993, p. 12.

20 Ibid., p. 10.

21 Xu Xiangcai, *Traditional Chinese Health Secrets*, YMAA Publication Centre, 2001, p. 10.

22 *Clin Ortho Related Res*, 1980, 152: 35, from Kitty Champion, 'Dial M for Milk', *What Doctors Don't Tell You*, 5(1).

23 H. M. Taggart and S. E. Connor, 'The Relation of Exercise Habits to Health Beliefs and Knowledge about Osteoporosis', *Journal of American College Health*, 44, 1995, pp. 127–30.

24 Since China has become more Westernized there are an increasing number of people with weight problems.

25 L. H. Kushi, E. B. Lenart and W. C. Willett, 'Health Implications of a Mediterranean Diet in the Light of Contemporary Knowledge of Meat, Wine, Fats and Oil', *American Journal of Clinical Nutrition*, 61, 1995, pp. 1416S–27S.

26 K. Godfrey et al., 'Maternal Nutrition in Early and Late Pregnancy in Relation to Placental and Fetal Growth', *British Medical Journal*, 17 February 1996.

27 Chinese Medicine practitioners look at the tongue when making a diagnosis. The tongue should be a healthy pale-red colour and a pale tongue can indicate that a person has Blood deficiency.

28 For more information on food combinations read F. M. Lappé, *Diet for a Small Planet*, Ballantyne, 1978.

29 Verbal communication from Francis Blake, Standards Director, Soil Association, February 2008.

30 *Living Earth*, No. 188, October 1995. For more information contact Soil Association, South Plaza, Marlborough Street, Bristol BS1 3NX, tel: 0117 314 5000, website: www.soilassociation.org.

31 Verbal communication from Francis Blake, Standards Director, Soil Association, February 2008.

32 Ibid.

33 G. Young, *The Wisdom of the Chinese Kitchen*, Simon and Schuster, 1999, pp. 20–1.

34 A. Hicks, *Principles of Chinese Medicine*, Thorsons, 1996.

35 Xu Xinagcai *Traditional Chinese Health Secrets*, YMAA Publication Centre, Boston MA, 2001, p. 13.

36 M. Timlin, M. Pereira, M. Story and D. Neumark-Sztainer, 'Breakfast Eating and Weight Change in a 5-year Prospective Analysis of Adolescents: Project EAT (Eating Among Teens)', *Pediatrics*, 121(3), March 2008, pp. 638–645.

37   Enqin Zhang *Health Preservation and Rehabilitation*, Publishing House of Shanghai College of TCM, 1988, p. 100.

38   N. Taylor, *Green Tea, The Natural Secret for a Healthier Life*, Kensington Books, 1998, pp. 31–88.

39   Ibid.

40   Xu Xiangcai, *Traditional Chinese Health Secrets*, YMAA Publication Centre, Boston, MA, 2001, p. 17.

41   S. Mathias et al., 'Coffee, Plasma Cholesterol, and Lipoproteins: A Population Study in an Adult Community', *American Journal of Epidemiology*, 121(6), 1985, pp. 896–905.

42   D. N. Ugarriza, S. Klingner and S. O'Brien, 'Premenstrual Syndrome: Diagnosis and Intervention', *Nurse Practitioner*, 23(9), 1998, pp. 40, 45, 49–52; L. M. Dickerson, P. J. Mazyck and M. H. Hunter, 'Premenstrual Syndrome', *American Family Physician*, 67(8), 2003, pp. 1743–52; K. T. Barnhart, E. W. Freeman and S. J. Sondheimer, 'A Clinician's Guide to the Premenstrual Syndrome', *Medical Clinics of North America*, 79(6), 1995, pp. 1457–72.

43   R. Urgert et al., 'Heavy Coffee Consumption and Plasma Homocysteine: A Randomized Controlled Trial in Healthy Volunteers', *American Journal of Clinical Nutrition*, 72(5), 2000, pp. 1107–10.

44   Y. J. Park et al., 'Association of Diet with Menopausal Symptoms in Korean Middle-aged Women', *Taehan Kanho Hakhoe chi*, 33(3), 2003, pp. 386–94.

45   P. Happonen, S. Voutilainen and J. T. Salonen, 'Coffee Drinking is Dose-dependently Related to the Risk of Acute Coronary Events in Middle-aged Men', *Journal of Nutrition*, 134(9), 2004, pp. 2381–6.

46   J. D. Lane et al., 'Caffeine Effects on Cardiovascular and Neuroendocrine Responses to Acute Psychosocial Stress and their Relationship to Level of Habitual Caffeine Consumption', *Psychosomatic Medicine*, 52(3), 1990, pp. 320–36.

Chapter 4: Secrets to Balance Our Emotions

1   *Huang Qi Nei Jing* (*Yellow Emperor's Classic of Internal Medicine*). The book is in two parts, and this quotation is from the part called the 'Su Wen' or Simple Questions, Chapter 39. There are many translations.

2   G. Ironson et al., 'The Effects of Anger on Left Ventricular Fraction in Coronary Artery Disease', *American Journal of Cardiology*, 1992, pp. 281–5.

3   B. McEwen and E. Stellar, 'Stress and Metastasis', *Archives of Internal Medicine*, 27 September 1993, pp. 2093–101.

4   R. W. Bartrop et al., 'Depressed Lymphocyte Function after Bereavement', *Lancet*, 16 April 1977, pp. 834–7.

5   Identified by Elisabeth Kübler-Ross in her groundbreaking book *On Death and Dying,* Macmillan, 1969.

6   My thanks to Jane Serraillier for her reminder of this prayer.

7   Liu Zhengcai, *The Mystery of Longevity*, Foreign Languages Press, Beijing, 1990, p. 34.

8   A. Stone et al., 'Secretory IgA Antibody is Associated with Daily Mood', *Journal of Personality and Social Psychology*, 52, May 1987, pp. 988–93.

9   C. Peterson, M. Seligman and G. Vaillant, 'Pessimistic Explanatory Style is a Risk Factor for Physical Illness: A 35-year Longitudinal Study', *Journal of Personality and Social Psychology*, 55(1), 1988, pp. 23–7.

10 Liu Zhengcai, *The Mystery of Longevity*, Foreign Languages Press, Beijing, 1990, p. 32.

11 Hexagon 'Obstruction', *I Ching* (Book of Changes), trs. R. Wilhelm, Routledge and Kegan Paul, 1983, p. 152.

12 These perceptual positions were developed by Robert Dilts and are used in Neuro Linguistic Programming (NLP). For more on NLP, read J. O'Connor and I. McDermott, *The Principles of NLP*, Thorsons, 1996.

13 For more on Focusing, see E. Gendlin, *Focusing*, Rider Books, 2003; A. W. Cornell, *The Power of Focusing*, New Harbinger Publications, 1996.

14 My thanks to Barbara McGavin from the Bath Focusing Centre, UK, for her help describing the Focusing process.

15 There are many good Focusing websites, such as the Focusing Institute www.focusing.org; Focusing Resources www.focusingresources.com; British Focusing Teachers Association www.focusing.org.uk.

16 For more ways of reframing, see R. Bandler and J. Grinder, *Reframing*, Real People Press, 1983.

17 Linda Chih-Ling Koo, *Nourishment of Life*, Commercial Press, 1987, p. 111.

18 Verbal communication from Dr Shen Hongxun, a *qigong* and *tai chi chuan* teacher, in 1995.

19 Linda Chih-Ling Koo, *Nourishment of Life*, Commercial Press, 1987, p. 119.

Chapter 5: Secrets of Balancing Work, Rest and Exercise

1   *Tai ji quan* is also called *tai chi chuan* and *qigong* is also called *chi gung* – according to the different transliterations of the Chinese characters.

2   Although this kind of healthy routine is still followed by some of the younger Chinese generation it is more common among older Chinese people. Some of this has been lost with modernization.

3   'Objective Measurement of Levels and Patterns of Physical Activity', *Arch Dis Child*, Online First, 2007, doi: 10.1136/adc.2006.112136.

4 ME is short for *myalgic encephalomyelitis*, a post-viral syndrome. *'Myalgic'* means pain in the muscles and *'encephalomyelitis'* means inflammation of the brain and nerves. For more on post-viral syndromes, see p. 192.

5 L. Breslow and N. Breslow, 'Health Practises and Disability: Some Evidence from Alameda County', *Preventative Medicine*, 1993, pp. 86–95.

6 S. Chollar, 'Psychological Benefits of Exercise', *American Health*, June 1995.

7 H. M. Taggart and S. E. Connor, 'The Relation of Exercise Habits to Health Beliefs and Knowledge about Osteoporosis', *Journal of American College Health*, 44, November 1995.

8 T. W. Rowland, *Exercise and Children's Health*, Human Kinetics Books, 1989, p. 106.

9 Xu Xiangcai, *Traditional Chinese Health Secrets*, YMAA Publications Centre, 2001, p. 33.

10 *Medicine & Science in Sports & Exercise*, 28, 1996, pp. 1235–42.

11 J. E. Manson et al., 'A Prospective Study of Walking as Compared with Vigorous Exercise in the Prevention of Coronary Heart Disease in Women', *New England Journal of Medicine*, 341, 26 August 1999, pp. 650–8.

12 *International Journal of Obesity Related Metabolic Disorders*, 24, 2000, pp. 1303–9.

13 L. McTaggart, 'Walking Towards Fitness', *What Doctors Don't Tell You*, 18(11), February 2008; *Medicine & Science in Sports & Exercise*, 34, 2002, pp. 1468–74.

14 www.walking.about.com/od/healthbenefits/BenefitsofWalkingHowWalking ReducesHealthRisks.htm (search date 18 February 2008).

15 For more about these gates, see B. Frantzis, *Opening the Energy Gates of Your Body*, Blue Snake Books, 2006, p. 142.

16 My thanks to Bill Ryan of Toward Harmony for allowing me to use this 'more *qi* in your practice' tip. For more *Tai Chi* and *Qigong* tips about energy awareness and your personal exercise practice, see www.towardharmony.com.

17 Some of this is adapted from 'Ten Walking Mistakes to Avoid', www.walking.about. com/cs/beginners/a/10mistakes10.htm (search date 18 February 2008).

18 *Practical Ways to Good Health through Chinese Traditional Medicine*, China Reconstructs Press, Beijing, 1989.

19 R. Ornstein and D. Sobel, *Healthy Pleasures*, Addison Wesley, 1989, p. 120.

20 Xu Xiangcai, *Traditional Chinese Health Secrets*, YMAA Publication Centre, 2001, p. 21.

21 R. Ornstein and D. Sobel, *Healthy Pleasures*, Addison Wesley, 1989, p. 119.

22 *Science News*, 161(22), 1 June 2002, p. 341.

23 From the BBC news website www.news.bbc.co.uk/1/hi/magazine/7114661.stm (search date 2 February 2008).

24 Adapted from an exercise in *300 Questions on Qigong Exercises*, Guangdong Science and Technology Press, 1994, p. 67.

25 My thanks to Bill Ryan for allowing me to use this 'more *qi* in your practice' tip. For more tips about *qigong* practice, see www.towardharmony.com.

26 K. M. Sancier, *Anti Aging Benefits of Qigong*, Beijing, 1996, p. 147.

27 Ibid.

28 B. K. Frantzis, *Opening the Energy Gates of Your Body*, Blue Snake Books, 2006, p. 28.

29 My thanks to Bill Ryan for allowing me to use some of this 'more *qi* in your practice' tip. For more tips about *qigong* practice, see www.towardharmony.com.

30 B. K. Frantzis, *Opening the Energy Gates of Your Body*, Blue Snake Books, 2006, pp. 94–101.

31 For more on *qigong,* read B. K. Frantzis, *Opening the Energy Gates of Your Body*, Blue Snake Books, 2006.

32 Liu Zhengcai, *The Mystery of Longevity*, Foreign Languages Press, Beijing, 1990, p. 77.

33 Ibid, p. 55.

Chapter 6: Secrets to Protect Ourselves from the Environment

1 M. Gauquelin, *How Atmospheric Conditions Affect Your Health*, ASI Publishers, 1989, p. 62.

2 M. Kaiser, *How the Weather Affects Your Health*, Michelle Anderson Publishing, 2002, p. 26.

3 Microbes causing illness were first discovered in the West in the late 19th century!

4 M. Gauquelin, *How Atmospheric Conditions Affect Your Health*, ASI Publishers, 1989, p. 39.

5 Ibid, p. 99.

6 M. Kaiser, *How the Weather Affects Your Health*, Michelle Anderson Publishing, 2002, p. 72.

Chapter 8: Staying Healthy and Preventing Disease

1 For more information about asthma, see the British Lung Foundation website (www.lunguk.org).

2 For more information about this, see the British Acupuncture Council (BAcC) website (www.acupuncture.org.uk).

3 For more about diabetes, see Diabetes UK's website (www.diabetes.org.uk).

4 For more information, see www.acupuncture.org.uk/content/Library/doc/migraine_bp1.pdf (accessed 10 February 2008).

Glossary

Blood

Chinese medicine teaches that Blood nourishes and moistens the body and allows the Spirit to be settled and calm.

Blood deficiency

This is a general term used when the Blood is no longer able to carry out the functions listed above. Blood deficiency leads to symptoms such as dry skin, insomnia, dizziness, tinnitus, numbness, scanty periods, poor memory, a tendency to startle easily and anxiety. Symptoms specific to the organ which has become Blood deficient will also manifest.

Blood stagnation

This is a term used when the Blood is 'stuck' and unable to move properly. It can cause symptoms such as blood clots, purple veins and/or severe, fixed, stabbing pain.

Cold

A climatic cause of disease which can manifest with symptoms such as aversion to cold, cold limbs, contraction of the tendons, thin, watery, clear discharges and severe pain relieved by warmth and aggravated by cold.

Damp

A climatic cause of disease which can manifest with symptoms such as aversion to damp or humidity, heavy limbs, heavy head, no appetite, a stuffy feeling in the chest or stomach area, recurrent dirty discharges or secretions and/or depressions.

Dryness

A climatic cause of disease which can manifest with symptoms such as a dry throat, dry mouth, dry nose, dry lips, dry skin, dry stools and/or scanty urination.

Heart functions
Some important functions of the Heart are i) to 'house' the Spirit; and ii) to circulate the Blood.

Heat
A climatic cause of disease which can manifest with symptoms such as an aversion to heat, sweating, dark-scanty urine, headache, dry lips and thirst.

Kidney functions
Some important functions of the Kidneys are to i) store constitutional essence; and ii) to control the water functions in the body.

Liver functions
Some important functions of the Liver are to i) allow the *qi* to flow smoothly throughout the body; and ii) to 'store' the Blood.

Lung functions
Some important functions of the Lungs are to i) control our ability to breath and take in *qi* via the Lungs; and ii) to disperse defensive or *'wei' qi* to the skin, thus protecting us from the effects of the climate.

Phlegm
Phlegm arises from stagnation of the body fluids. It can cause symptoms such as mucous in the Lungs, nodules on joints, kidney or gall stones and/or lumps under the skin. If it blocks the Heart 'orifices' it can cause some forms of mental illness.

Qi
(Pronounced 'chi'.) Usually translated as 'energy'. *Qi* moves, transforms, protects, holds and warms everything in our body.

Qi deficiency
This is a general term used when the *qi* has become weak. When the *qi* is deficient it can no longer perform the functions listed above and symptoms of general weakness and tiredness will arise. Symptoms specific to the organ which has become deficient will also manifest.

Qi stagnation
This is a general term used when the *qi* is not moving properly. Because *qi* is very refined and light, *qi* stagnation will often come and go according to our

moods or with movement. It will cause many symptoms including ones which appear and disappear, distending pain which moves around, symptoms which are better with massage, mood swings and/or depression.

Spirit

The Chinese describe the Spirit as the part of us which is responsible for our overall sense of purpose and identity. A 'settled' Spirit also allows us to think clearly and have good concentration, memory and sleep.

Spleen functions

Some important functions of the Spleen are to i) transform and move food, drink and our thoughts; ii) to rule over all digestive functions; and iii) to keep the Blood in the blood vessels.

Stomach function

One important function of the Stomach is to digest or 'rot and ripen' food and drink.

Wind

A climatic cause of disease which can manifest as rapidly changing symptoms, symptoms which move around, symptoms which affect the top part of the body and ones which affect the Lung first. Other manifestations can be itching, tremors, convulsions and/or numbness.

Yang

More active energy. Some *yang* qualities are heat, dryness, movement and an upward direction.

Yin

More passive energy. Some *yin* qualities are coldness, wetness, stillness and sinking down.

Yin/yang balance

Yin and *yang* are opposites as well as constantly interacting. These two qualities balance each other. When out of balance they cause disharmony in the body, mind and spirit, leading to illness.

Reading list

Chih-Ling Koo, Linda (1987) *Nourishment of Life – Health in Chinese Society*, Hong Kong, The Commercial Press.

Flaws, Bob (1993) *Arisal of the Clear – A Simple Guide to Healthy Eating According to Traditional Chinese Medicine*, Blue Poppy Press.

Flaws, Bob (1994) *Imperial Secrets of Health and Longevity*, Blue Poppy Press.

Frantzis, Bruce Kumar (1998) *Relaxing into Your Being*, North Atlantic Books.

Frantzis, Bruce Kumar (2006) *Opening the Energy Gates of Your Body*, Blue Snake Books.

Gendlin, Eugene (2003) *Focusing*, Rider Books.

Hicks, Angela (2010) *The Acupunture Handbook*, Piatkus.

Hicks, Angela and John (1999) *Healing Your Emotions*, London, Thorsons.

Housheng, Lin and Peiyu, Luo (1982) *Three Hundred Questions on Qigong Exercises*, Guangdong Science and Technology Press.

Kaiser, M. (2002) *How the Weather Affects your Health*, Michele Anderson Publishing.

Leggett, Daverick (1997) *Helping Ourselves*, Meridian Press.

Leggett, Daverick (1999) *Recipes for Self Healing*, Meridian Press.

McDermott, Ian and O'Connor, Joseph (2001) *NLP and Health*, London, Thorsons.

Ornstein, Robert and Sobel, David (1989) *Healthy Pleasures*, Addison Wesley.

Qingnan, Zeng (2002) *Methods of Traditional Chinese Health Care*, Beijing, Foreign Languages Health.

Various Chinese authors (1989) *Practical Ways to Good Health through Traditional Chinese Medicine*, China Reconstructs Press.

Weiser Cornell, Ann (1996) *The Power of Focusing – A Practical Guide to Emotional Self-healing*, New Harbinger Publications.

Xiangcai, Xu (2001) *Traditional Chinese Health Secrets*, YMAA Publication Centre.

Young, Grace (1999) *The Wisdom of the Chinese Kitchen*, Simon & Schuster.

Zhengcai, Lui (1999) *The Mystery of Longevity*, Beijing, Foreign Languages Press.

Useful addresses

If you wish to find an acupuncturist or Chinese herbalist in the UK, contact the following professional bodies:

Acupuncture
British Acupuncture Council
63 Jeddo Road
London W12 9HQ
Tel: 020 8735 0400
Website: www.acupuncture.org.uk
E-mail: info@acupuncture.org.uk

Herbs
The Register of Chinese Herbal Medicine
Office 5
1 Exeter Street
Norwich NR2 4QB
Tel: 01603 623994
Website: www.rchm.co.uk
Email: herbmed@rchm.co.uk

To contact the author
College of Integrated Chinese Medicine
19 Castle Street
Reading
Berkshire RG4 7TQ
Tel: 0118 9508880
Website: www.cicm.org.uk
Email: admin@cicm.org.uk

Index